Lean 51

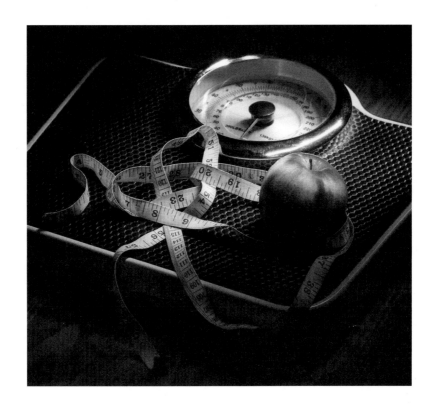

By Dr. Gregory Oliver

LEAN 51

Dear New LEAN Team Member:

You have made a great decision! Congratulations on taking the first step on a journey that will take you to improved health, incredible energy, and an enhanced lifestyle. You have spent too much time living in a body that is over-fat. You know that every day you have quietly wished to be lean. Your health is being adversely affected and the excess weight creates problems in many areas of your life.

Now it's time to leave this past behind you. The choice you made to start the LEAN 51 Program can have dramatic positive effects on your life. I have seen this happen over and over for people on the LEAN 51 weight management system. Our patients and clients tell me how energetic they feel and how excited they are for each day's new experiences. Being lean not only adds years to your life, but will create a new level of personal power and self-confidence that you may not have experienced before. Knowing that you are in control and that you are committed to a more healthful lifestyle raises your standards in all areas of your life.

You will find the LEAN 51 Program to be simple and straight forward. There are no gimmicks or quick fixes, but your weight loss will be rapid and sustained. Following the Ten Step plan each day will create a new habit of eating well and will teach your body to be a fat-burning machine.

LEAN 51 is not a fad diet. It is a plan designed from years of patient care, study of the weight loss industry, and my personal experience with weight loss. I have evaluated and reviewed dozens of dietary programs. Though other programs may be sound, I have expanded on what I feel are some of the best aspects of several programs and incorporated these beneficial components along with new proven techniques into our own simple, step-by-step daily guide to fat reduction. This makes LEAN 51 a powerful tool for anyone desiring to lose the fat and become healthy.

The LEAN 51 Kit provides everything you need to immediately start on the program. I advise scanning through the guidebook first to become familiar with it. Follow the Ten Step Pattern and you will be on your way to Living Lean, Living Long, and Living Life.

I wish you well as you begin your journey toward living lean... The LEAN 51 Way!

Dr. Greg Oliver

Founder, LEAN 51

Contents

Introduction to LEAN 51

Quick Start Guide

KEY POINTS:

- QUICK WEIGHT LOSS: Average weight loss is up to 15 pounds a month
- GREAT TASTE: Portion Controlled Snack-meals are extremely satisfying
- SIMPLE PLAN: Eat every 2 ½ - 3 hours
- '51': 5 Snack-meals a day; 1 Healthy (Lean and Green) meal a day
- NO HUNGER: Eating every 2 ½-3 hours eliminates cravings and hunger
- SUPPORT: Physician and Health Coach support through our website and email
- COST: Lower cost than other programs, and less than or equal to your current food costs per month

Healthy Meal Options

Protein: 4-6 oz. servings

Grilled, baked, broiled, or poached – not fried.

Fish	Chicken	Egg Whites	98% Lean Cold Cuts
Shellfish	Lean Beef	Egg Beaters	Tuna
Game Meats	Lamb	Veggie Burgers	Fat Free Cheese
Turkey	Lean Pork Cuts	Tofu	Low Fat Cottage Cheese

Vegetables: 2 servings (up to 2 cups total)

Celery	Cabbage	Broccoli	Carrots
Cucumber	Mushrooms	Asparagus	Scallions
Lettuce	Peppers	Tomatoes	Onions
Spinach	Radishes	Okra	Squash
Greens	Sprouts	Turnips	Kale
Cauliflower	Eggplant	Green beans	Mixed Veggies/ Salad

Condiments: Small amounts of mustard, ketchup, dill pickle, and most herbal and natural seasonings may be used.

Healthy Fats: 2 Tablespoons of regular or low-carb dressing
1 Teaspoon of margarine
1 Tablespoon of Olive Oil

Beverages: Drink 80 oz. of water plus limited zero calorie liquids

---

1
Healthy Meal

4-6 oz. Lean Protein
2 Vegetable Servings
*Typically lunch or dinner.

5
Snack Meal

Choose From:
Portion Controlled Protein Bars, Shakes, Puddings, Soups, Crunch Bars, Fruit Drinks, and many more available Snack Meals.

Eat one of your 6 meals every 2 ½ - 3 hours

"What we prepare for is what we shall get."
~William Graham Sumner

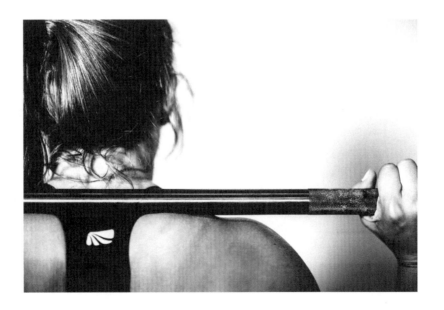

"Change your thoughts and you change your world"

~Norman Vincent Peale

Introduction to LEAN 51

I was a fat doctor. How can a doctor tell his patients to lose weight and get healthy if he can't?

In February of 2002, on a typical Thursday morning, I stepped into the exam room to see my next patient, Natalie. I had been Natalie's physician for over 15 years and she was 87 years of age. When I shook her hand and asked her how she was, she stopped, stared, and said, "Doc, you're fat." Stunned and embarrassed, I agreed with her and moved on to assist her in taking care of her medical needs that day. Her comment stayed with me all day and bothered me like a rough tag in the collar of my too-tight shirt.

It was true; my athletic build from high school and college sports days was gone. I was 5'10" tall and 218 lb. I calculated I was 43-lbs. overweight. I was obese by my own medical definition. The next day, I was attending a conference and met some physicians who had been successful helping patients lose fat and reach their optimal weight. I studied their program and reviewed many of the current programs on the market. After this research period, I concluded that a dietary plan, which incorporated proteins, carbohydrates, and fats in appropriate combinations, would be the healthiest. I developed my plan with many new concepts and techniques and started on my own "Lean Program." In five months I lost 42-lbs.

So many people wanted to know what I had done to lose the weight, that I began giving seminars and building a team of people who were committed to Living Lean, Living Long, and Living Life. The LEAN 51 Program is an enhanced protein, reduced carbohydrate, controlled fat dietary regimen. It does not eliminate any component of good sound nutrition. Join me and thousands of others. I know you can do it. Natalie knows you can too!

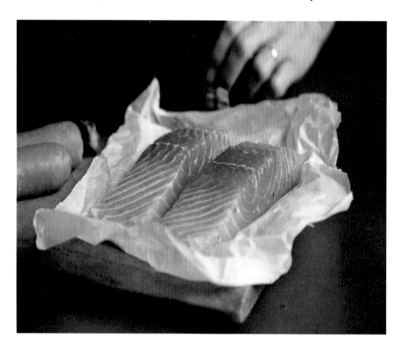

Why LEAN 51

Health – A state of physical, mental, and emotional well-being.

Over the last 30 years, I have dealt with sickness, disease, injury, and death as a family doctor. I have also been actively involved in disease prevention, wellness, and health maintenance. I calculate that I have sat in the exam room, listened to and evaluated approximately 300,000 people. This experience has led me to believe that it is the desire of all individuals to feel good and live as long as possible, providing they have their health. Yet, day after day my patients, and 80% of all Americans, live an unhealthy lifestyle that will most definitely shorten their lives. They are overweight. More precisely, they are over fat.

My overweight and obese patients routinely feel tired, weak, short of breath, and generally bad. Many have Type II Diabetes, premature heart disease, joint pain, sleeping problems, and are poorly conditioned to meet the demands of our stressful world. In the past, this gloomy scenario was not well-managed by my profession. Now there is the LEAN 51 Program. Reduction of fat and achieving a leaner body weight can have dramatic effects on your overall health, physical fitness, endurance, and improve mental and emotional well-being.

What is so important about starting LEAN 51? An extensive review of the medical literature reveals that there are several factors, which lead to a long, healthy life. People who live into their 80's and beyond have been found to follow certain lifestyle patterns. Interestingly enough, all of these factors are under our control. These "Long Life" factors are as follows:

1. Maintaining lean body weight
2. Avoiding cigarettes
3. Exercising regularly
4. Having strong social relationships
5. Having good coping skills
6. Learning new things regularly

This manual and the LEAN 51 program focuses on #1 and #3 – maintaining lean body weight and exercising regularly. The people who live the longest are lean and eat a balanced diet of lean source proteins, fruits and vegetables, and perform moderate daily physical activity. The LEAN 51 program promotes and teaches this lifestyle. That is why we say "Live Lean, Live Long, and Live Life."

If you want to enjoy life to the fullest, and live as long as you were intended to live, then you have started on the right path by beginning the LEAN 51 Plan. Get excited about turning your life in the direction of health and fitness.

How Much Should I Weigh

There are several ways to decide what your ideal body weight should be. The first thing I recommend is to be totally honest with yourself. No more claims about being "big boned" or coming from a family of large people. Your lean or ideal weight is the weight you should be at to live the longest and feel the best. For some, you may feel great within 10 pounds of that weight. That's OK. We are not doing this to create a team of gaunt-looking, underweight models. We want you to be at your optimum health and weight.

The BMI (Body Mass Index) is a good guide for determining your health risk. The BMI is a calculation of a person's weight in relation to their height. Once a person reaches their adult height, the BMI will only change when weight is either gained or lost. The BMI correlates very well with risk of disease caused from being overweight. Medical professionals, including your doctor, feel a BMI of 22 is optimal for good health.

A BMI of 25 to 29.9 is considered overweight and implies an increased risk of disease. Obesity is diagnosed with a BMI of 30 or greater and marked (morbid) obesity is present at a BMI of 40 and above. There is a problem with using the BMI for a person with low body fat and high muscle mass. This person is still in good health but the BMI will show a high number due to the increased weight of the muscle tissue. If possible it is best to get a body composition measurement to determine not only weight, but total body fat, water, and lean tissue percentages. Unless you work out regularly and have significant muscle mass above normal, the BMI will be a good guide to work with in determining your health risk.

Calculate your current BMI. Consult the BMI chart on the next page. Find your height in inches along the left side of the chart. Move across the chart to the right to find your weight. You can also use this chart to find your ideal body weight or a weight that puts you in the healthy zone. Another simple method to determine lean body weight is to use the following formula:

Women - At 5-ft tall should weigh 100 pounds, add 5 pounds for each inch taller.
Men - At 5-ft tall should weigh 106 pounds, add 6 pounds for each inch taller.

Now you know what your optimum weight should be for your height. When you know where you're at, you can develop a roadmap to where you're going. So get out the map, start the motor, shift into gear, and get lean.

Body Mass Index (BMI)

Height	Weight (in pounds)																
	19	20	21	22	23	24	25	26	27	28	29	30	31	32	33	34	35
4'10"	91	96	100	105	110	115	119	124	129	134	138	143	148	153	158	162	167
4'11"	94	99	104	109	114	119	124	128	133	138	143	148	153	158	163	168	173
5'	97	102	107	112	118	123	128	133	138	143	148	153	158	163	168	174	179
5'1"	100	106	111	116	122	127	132	137	142	148	153	158	164	169	174	180	185
5'2"	104	109	115	120	126	131	136	142	147	153	158	164	169	175	180	186	191
5'3"	107	113	118	124	130	135	141	146	152	158	163	169	175	180	186	191	197
5'4"	110	116	122	128	134	140	145	151	157	163	169	174	180	186	192	197	204
5'5"	114	120	126	132	138	144	150	156	162	168	174	180	186	192	198	204	210
5'6"	118	124	130	136	142	148	155	161	167	173	179	186	192	198	204	210	216
5'7"	121	127	134	140	146	153	159	166	172	178	185	191	198	204	211	218	223
5'8"	125	131	137	144	151	157	164	171	177	184	190	197	203	210	216	223	230
5'9"	128	135	142	149	155	162	169	176	182	189	196	203	209	216	223	230	236
5'10"	132	139	146	153	160	167	174	181	188	195	202	209	216	222	229	236	243
5'11"	136	146	150	157	165	172	179	186	193	200	208	215	222	229	235	243	250
6'	140	147	154	162	169	177	184	191	199	206	213	221	228	235	242	250	258
6'1"	144	151	159	166	174	182	189	197	204	212	219	227	235	242	250	258	265
6'2"	148	155	163	171	179	186	194	202	210	218	225	233	241	249	256	264	272
6'3"	152	160	168	176	184	192	200	208	216	224	232	240	248	256	264	272	279

BMI Below 25
Healthy weight

BMI 25-30
Overweight

BMI 30+
Obese

"Before you begin a thing, remind yourself that difficulties and delays quite impossible to foresee are ahead...You can only see one thing clearly, and that is your goal. Form a mental vision of that and cling to it through thick and thin."

~Kathleen Norris

Take a Picture / Paint a Portrait

Before starting on the LEAN 51 Program, take a few minutes to establish goals. What do you want to accomplish with the LEAN 51 Program? Complete the exercise below before going any further. This will help you to understand the reasons you want to change your lifestyle and be the best and healthiest you can be.

YOUR PERSONAL PICTURE

Take a mental picture of your current health by writing down the answers to these questions.

- What is my current weight? _____
- What is my current dress/pant size? _____
- Do I get tired easily? _____
- Do I have sleeping problems? _____
- Do I get short of breath easily? _____
- Can I keep up with others physically? _____
- Do my friends and family worry about my weight? _____
- Do I take medicines for high blood pressure, diabetes or high cholesterol?_____
- Do I have back pain, knee pain, or foot pain?_____
- Do I avoid getting my picture taken? _____
- Am I comfortable at the beach or pool? _____
- Do I fit into seats in theaters, airplanes, or amusement rides comfortably?_____

Write down anything else that currently concerns you about your weight and health.

This exercise is not designed to focus on negative things. It is intended to take an honest look at where you are right now. This will help you in the following exercise to decide what type of body, health, and level of fitness you desire compared to your current state of health. When you complete this process, you will have a clear image of the gap between where you are now and where you want to be. It is the gap we are going to close as we work together on your LEAN 51 Program.

OUR SPLENDID PORTRAIT

Now, paint a beautiful mental portrait of how you want your health to be. Review these statements about your potential future self. Add other statements you want to describe the future you. Write out all of the descriptive phrases that describe you. Do this in the first-person tense, i.e. "I look years younger at my lean weight."

- I am full of energy now.
- I look years younger at my lean weight.
- My new clothes fit great, they don't bind or pull.
- I feel stronger and physically fit.
- Theater, stadium and airplane seats are comfortable now.
- My family and friends are proud of me and are following my lead to a healthier lifestyle.
- Sleep is easier and more restful.
- I have a strong sense of accomplishment and much healthier self-esteem.
- I breathe easy as I climb stairs and perform physical tasks.
- I have a decreased chance of cancer and heart disease.
- My blood pressure, cholesterol and blood sugars are in control and at healthy levels.
- My relationships with others are improved and my romantic life is "spicing" up.
- I'm on my way to a longer, healthier life.
- I am Living Lean, Living Long, and Living Life!

Do not skip this session! This exercise is a critical part of your long-term weight management program. Writing a detailed description of how you want to live will assist your subconscious to help you make better decisions every minute, every hour and every day. See who you can become. Read your personal statement every day. Picture yourself as you read it. Become so familiar with the new you that you mentally reach your goal well before you're your body gets there. You will begin to live the Lean Lifestyle as you work toward your ultimate goal.

This visualization exercise will be revisited as part of the goal setting step in the Ten Step Program section. As you progress through the Ten Step Program chapter, repeat this visualization process again to deeply establish the images in your mind. When you can visualize your future vividly and easily, you will have the mental power to stay the course. We know that seeing is believing; but, in this case, believing will lead to seeing.

I see you as a lean, fit, strong, healthy individual, who is an example to everyone around you, and that living the life you desire is simply a matter of choices, vision, and persistence. You have it within you. Now, paint your new life portrait and live it each day.

"Knock the 't' off the can't."

~ George Reeves

Increase Body Motion

I routinely ask my patients, "How much physical activity do you get?" The answer given by someone who is lean is very different from the answer given by an overweight patient. The fit or lean person will tell me specifically what type of exercise they perform and exactly how often and for how long they work at it. An example might be – "I walk 45 minutes 5 days a week." By contrast, my overweight patients answer the question by saying "I'm very busy all day long." I've learned "being busy" doesn't burn extra calories.

Getting up early, driving to work, stopping by the fast food window, sitting at a desk with lots of paperwork or computer work, picking up the kids from school and delivering them to soccer, piano lessons, Boy Scouts, cheerleading, etc., racing home to prepare a fast meal, crashing on the couch to catch a couple of sit-coms or reality shows, is not physical activity.

When this is explained to them and I inform them what real physical activity consists of, I'm often told that there is no time in their busy schedule for that type of activity. We all have choices to make. We all have 24 hours in each day. If you are serious about living a healthier, longer, and more satisfying life, you must make time for physical activity.

I understand it is not practical to go from a lifestyle of no exercise to 30-40 minutes of exercise a day. I recommend starting very slowly and gradually building up your physical activity. If you do what many people who haven't exercised in years do, which is starting too fast and too intensely, I will be seeing you in my office with an injury. Starting at your own baseline is a smart place to begin.

Each of us walk every day. Some of us take a limited amount of steps, while others walk miles during their daily routine. I recommend a step tracking device. These devices count your steps as you move. Your goal is to find out how many steps you currently take in a normal day and then establish new goals to achieve. This enhancement in the amount of body motion will help you develop a long-term habit of increased physical activity and prevent the return of those unwanted pounds which you worked off in your LEAN 51 Program.

Wear the step tracking device every day and record the number of steps you take each day on the LEAN 51 tracker log. You don't have to join a gym or club to do this. You don't need special equipment to do this. You can walk indoors, outdoors, or on a treadmill. A specific walking program is suggested on the following pages to assist you in getting started and in increasing your motion. Your body was made to move. Increased movement will not only assist in losing fat, but it will aid your digestion, your immune system and your attitude.

You won't believe what you've been missing out on. Put on the tracking device and get started today. An added benefit is that wearing the device is a great conversation starter. Everyone wants to learn what type it is. Just tell them it's part of your journey to thin.

WALKING PROGRAM

Your ultimate goal will be 10,000 steps each day. Don't PANIC! This is your ultimate goal. Only after losing fat and eating better will you be able to reach this milestone. Now, relax and follow the steps listed below.

Step 1: How many steps do I take each day at the start of my LEAN 51 Program? To find this out, wear your step tracker each day for 1 week and record the daily total.

Monday   # _____ steps

Tuesday   # _____ steps

Wednesday # _____ steps

Thursday   # _____ steps

Friday   # _____ steps

Saturday   # _____ steps

Sunday   # _____ steps

Week 1 Total   _____ steps

Divide by 7 = my average steps per day at program start are _____. This is your baseline number.

Don't increase your activity above your usual level during this week.

Step 2: Set a new goal for week 2, week 3, week 4 and so on until you reach 10,000 steps a day. Use the chart to set these goals.

If your Baseline is:	Week: 1	2	3	4	5	6	Main. Goal
<2,000	2,500	3,250	4,000	5,000	6,000	7,500	10,000
3,000	3,500	4,250	5,500	7,000	8,000	10,000	10,000
4,000	4,500	5,250	6,250	7,500	8,500	10,000	10,000
5,000	5,500	6,250	7,000	8,000	9,000	10,000	10,000
6,000	6,500	7,000	8,000	9,000	10,000	11,000	11,000
7,000	7,500	8,000	9,000	10,000	11,000	12,000	12,000
8,000	8,500	9,000	10,000	11,000	12,000	13,000	13,000
9,000	9,500	10,000	11,000	12,000	13,000	14,000	14,000
10,000	10,500	11,000	12,000	13,000	14,000	15,000	15,000

These suggestions will help you increase your physical activity slowly and safely. You may modify this approach if you have physical or medical problems or you may increase the timetable if you are young and have no health issues. If you have questions, send us an e-mail at fatdocthindoc@gmail.com. We'll be happy to help you establish walking goals.

The LEAN 51 Ten Step Program

By closely following these 10 steps and by using the workbook as a detailed day-by-day guide, you will increase the effectiveness of this program and have greater success.

1. **Define Your Goals/Define your Future** – Focus on your future. Each day write and define your goals. Be specific. Be detailed. Be positive.
2. **Read the LEAN 51 Workbook** – Every day, read the lesson, fill-in the tracker form, write your goals, and use the journal to express your thoughts and feelings.
3. **Follow the LEAN 51 Menu Plan** – The menu is simple and straight forward. To lose weight, you must follow the plan exactly as written. Do not delete or substitute. This will adversely affect your weight loss.
4. **Use the LEAN 51 Daily Tracker** – Each day comes with a tracker form in the workbook. Extra forms may be copied as you cycle through the plan. Be honest with yourself as you fill it out.
5. **Eat Your Snack-meals** – Snack-meals Block Cravings – The snack-meals were specially chosen to go with the program. They will eliminate cravings and provide balanced nutrition throughout the day. They taste great!
6. **Take the Supplements Daily** – Take your Vitamin Supplements daily as directed. These packs include therapeutic vitamins, enzymes for digestion, and phytonutrients for overall health improvement.
7. **Drink Fluids** – Drink at least 80-oz. of non-caloric fluid daily. Use pure water, and limited non-caloric tea, coffee and zero calorie soft drink beverages. Limit caffeine to 1 or two cups daily. Taking your fluids will prevent dehydration and assist the fat-burning process.
8. **Increase Movement/Use a Step-Tracking Device** – Wear the tracker every day. Set weekly goals to increase your walking. The increase in physical activity will accelerate your weight loss and enhance your muscle tone. This habit will be important in your weight maintenance phase.
9. **Check Your Attitude** – Motivation is an inside job. Be sure to start each day with a positive attitude. Be grateful for what you have and every achievement you make.
10. **Stay in Touch** – Use e-mail to link yourself to the Team. Questions, encouragement, and celebration can be shared this way. Our staff will communicate with you and help coach you in this way. Use fatdocthindoc@gmail.com to reach us.

1. Define Your Goals – Define Your Future

If you are an American, there is an 80% chance that you are overweight. Statistics vary slightly, but it is generally accepted that 35% of adults in the U.S. are obese. Obesity is defined as a BMI greater than 30. Ideal weight is based on height and gender. A simple calculation can let you know what your ideal weight should be. If you are a woman, and you are 5 feet tall, your lean weight is 100 pounds. For every inch over 5 feet tall, add 5 pounds.

Example:
5'1" = 105 Pounds
5'2" = 110 Pounds

If you are male, and you are 5 feet tall, you should weigh 106 pounds. Add 6 pounds for every inch over 5 feet tall.

Example:
5'5" = 136 pounds
5'10" = 165 pounds
6'0" = 176 pounds

This calculation will get you very close to your ideal or lean body weight. I discussed Body Mass Index (BMI) and the BMI chart in the previous section. The BMI chart will give you another method to find your ideal healthy weight.

ow that you know what your ideal weight should be, it's time to establish goals. OK! you say, I've done this all before and never reached or maintained my goal weight. There is a very good reason that this has happened to you. Your goal was just a number. It had no emotional meaning to you. In fact, most of us see our ideal weight and instantly go into denial or depression. I used to blame the charts, saying there is no way people could live at that ridiculously low weight. I was very sure my "bone structure" wouldn't allow it. These were _excuses_ and rationalizations, which I call "rational lies." I focused on what it would take to be at that weight and not the positive consequences of living at that weight. When we think about the effort of dieting, the change required, the perceived pain involved, or the process itself, we unlock the negative in our mind.

Our subconscious doesn't like us to be in a bad or negative situation and moves us as fast as possible out of it. Therefore, we decide not to change our eating habits and the result is no weight loss. Just think about this – Tony Robbins once said... "the first three letters of the word diet are D-I-E." I don't think any of us want that – do we?

Let's look at goal setting in a different way. I want you to go through an exercise with me (the non-sweating kind). Get a pad of paper and a pencil or pen. Sit down in a quiet room. This process may require anywhere from 10 – 30 minutes.

At the top left of the page, I want you to write down your current weight. You don't have to share this with anyone. It's for your eyes only. At the top right corner of the paper write down your ideal weight based on the previous calculation you made. The difference between these numbers could be a few stubborn pounds or double to triple your ideal weight, or anywhere in between. Don't fret! My team and I are here to help you, one step at a time.

The next step may be difficult for some, but I assure you it will become easy over time. With your eyes closed, I want you to take a mental picture of your life at your current weight. Picture how you look. Picture how your friends and family see you. How do your clothes fit? How much energy do you have? Are you tired in your picture? Are you being treated for high blood pressure, diabetes, joint pain, back pain, bowel problems, or other overweight-related disorders? Can you play with your kids or grand-kids without getting winded? Can you get on the floor and back up? Picture your last visit to the pool or beach. Are you wearing a swimsuit or a cover-up? Do you fit comfortably in the seats at the theater, the arena, the stadium or an airplane? Do you snore or have sleep apnea?

Does this picture of yourself tell you it's time to change? I hope you have taken time to take this picture of your current life. I know we avoid photographs when we are overweight and certainly prefer not to see pictures of our overweight selves. This, however, is a mental picture of your current lifestyle. Now, take some time and write down how you pictured yourself. Answer some of the questions I posed to you. This may seem negative, yet it is this current picture that we want our mind to move away from. Take as much time and write as much as you need to fully describe your current weight-related concerns, difficulties, and struggles.

Now get up from the table or chair and move about. Clear you mind for a few minutes. Next, you are going to create a vision of life at your new lean body weight. Sit again, close your eyes, and this time I want you to paint a portrait of how you will live your life at your optimum weight. What do you look like in your portrait? How do you feel? Are you energetic and light on your feet? Your joints don't hurt. Your back is strong and pain free all day long. Your clothes are smaller and loose on your body.

People are amazed at how you look. Your doctor is proud of you and is most likely reducing or eliminating medications. Your life expectancy has increased and you are a healthful example to your family, your friends, and your acquaintances. You have all new clothes since the old ones don't fit. Your relationships are improving because your self-confidence is soaring. You wake up each day refreshed and excited in your body. You're ready to try new things. Many people, who know you, want you to help them get lean. We are all so very proud of you.

This portrait of you is a masterpiece and you created it. You are destined to Live Lean, Live long, and Live Life to the fullest. Write down, in detail, the specific image you had of yourself as you went through the portrait painting mental exercise. Put down on paper what you expect your life to be like when you are living at your lean body weight. You may want to write about your new life using lists, or you may write a narrative of your new lifestyle. Take your time and complete this exercise. It is important that your mind understand and permanently lock onto this image of the new you.

As you move through the LEAN 51 Manual on the pages ahead, you will be asked to write your goals each day. You might feel that this is redundant; however, success coach, Brian Tracey, has used this method with hundreds of thousands of people and found the daily goal writing exercise is a key for anyone truly desiring accomplishment in any area of their life. Use this technique to ingrain your goals and vision of your new lean self deeply into your brain. You will not fail. You will succeed. You will reach your goal and stay there.

2. Read the LEAN 51 Manual

I bet you are a diet expert. Anyone who is or has been overweight is a diet expert. You know about fat. You know about carbs. You know about exercise. You know all of the diet drugs.

You know everything there is to know about weight loss except how to make it happen permanently. I was also there and I am a doctor.

Be open to new ideas and learn how to permanently change your life. There is no magic. There is no special pill or drug. There is no miracle new breakthrough to melt you down to your ideal weight. The LEAN 51 program is a safe, sensible, step-by-step, day-by-day guide to assist you in becoming the person you envisioned in your portrait.

The manual should be reviewed prior to getting started. Then go back to Day One and begin on a date that you have set as your LEAN 51 Launch Day. Complete all the exercises and, when requested, use this manual as your personal how-to text book to achieve a life of optimal health.

EXERCISE:

- Put a picture of yourself as you are before starting the program on your Day 1 goal page.
- Send a picture of yourself before starting the program to me at our email: Fatdocthindoc@gmail.com.

3. Follow the LEAN 51 Daily Menu Plan

Some people like to follow instructions and some people don't. I don't. As I began this program, I made a decision that the goal I had painted in my mental portrait was more important than altering the menu. So, I followed the menu. You will find the LEAN 51 Program has a very simple menu plan. It is simple to use and has a wide variety of choices. You will not be hungry, because, you will eat 6 times daily. You eat real food from the grocery or at restaurants for your healthy meal and there are no special or fancy preparation requirements.

The menu will take you through the entire program. The program will kick start your body's ability to burn fat and will put your body into mild ketosis. Ketosis is safe and is nothing more than a biochemical sign our body is using fat as a source of energy. The ketones in our blood that cause ketosis are actually fuel derived from fat breakdown. The menu outlines exactly what to eat to begin to burn off the fat.

Lipolysis is the process of fat burning. While burning fat, the menu provides a specified amount of protein, carbohydrates, and fat to assist in safe, rapid fat loss and subsequent weight loss.

When you have reached your optimum weight and you match the portrait of health you mentally created, you will enter the maintenance part of your program.

In summary, the LEAN 51 menu plan is designed to get you off to a great start, promote healthy and consistent weight loss, allow for steady control of your metabolic rate, and give you the tools to maintain your optimal body weight for life.

4. Fill Out the Daily LEAN 51 Tracker Form

As I said earlier, we all know how to lose weight and eat right. In order to actually do it, we must record what we eat. The LEAN 51 Tracker is a simple check-off form to insure that you have eaten enough of the correct foods each day. This program is not about depriving yourself of food. It's about eating the right foods at the right time to accelerate your body's own fat-burning mechanisms.

As I have counseled LEAN 51 participants, I find that anytime someone is not losing weight, it is because they have reverted to that old "diet" program in their brain that tells them "less food is better." In the LEAN 51 program, you must eat approximately every 3 hours to increase your weight loss. Depending on your initial weight and the amount of weight you need to lose, we can advise you on any modifications to the plan. Remember, eat every 3 hours. Consider this when people ask you how you lost your weight. You can tell them you lost your weight while eating all day. Sounds crazy, but it is working for many people.

Even though each day of this manual has a Tracker Form, you might want to make extra copies and place them in a binder or folder to have on hand. You can transfer the day's data into the manual later, if desired. Some people prefer to keep the manual with them at all times. Be sure to check off everything you eat. This will help us to assist you as you progress through the program. Just trying to remember what you eat in your mind is a prescription for failure. If it's worth doing right, then it's worth writing down.

Tracking your actions will make it simpler to lose the weight, get healthy, and live longer.

5. Eat your Snack Meals – Snack Meals Block Cravings

I call the snack meals the magic of LEAN 51. It was hard for me to believe that I could eat every 3 hours and still lose weight, but I experienced it first-hand. I never got hungry. I remained satisfied throughout each day, and at times felt like I was eating too much and too often.

The reason that most diets fail is that dieters go into "diet mode" of deprivation. Just remember that every time you've gone on a diet, you had to muster up all your strength to cut out everything you wanted to eat so you could starve away 10-15 pounds only to become so hungry that you blew the diet and gained the weight back. If you can't keep from getting hungry, you'll never stay on a diet plan long enough to lose weight. Be sure to eat the snack-meals as outlined in the plan.

The snack-meals provided by the LEAN 51 Program have been selected because of their taste, nutrition, and compliance with the LEAN 51 formula. There are many bars and drinks available on the open market, but we have not seen the same success when randomly purchased items are used. Don't ever be caught without your snack-meals. Forgetting to eat every 3 hours will leave you hungry and may tempt you to eat food items not on the menu.

Warning you to be sure to eat every 3 hours throughout the day sounds contrary to what you've heard for years, but you can eat your way to a new healthy lifestyle. I know it works. You will know it soon.

6. Take Supplements Daily

Every day, people ask me, as their physician, if they need vitamins and supplements. I tell them that if they eat a well-balanced diet, get plenty of rest, are at their lean weight, don't smoke cigarettes or drink excess alcohol, and have no stress; they don't need any vitamin supplements. The point is that everybody needs a therapeutic multi-vitamin supplement, proper digestive enzymes, and in a low fish-eating country like the U.S., a balanced Omega-3 fatty acid supplement is necessary. The LEAN 51 Program provides those essential elements.

As with the snack-meals, we have found some of the best vitamins and Omega-3 fatty acids on the market and have made them part of the LEAN 51 Program. Unfortunately, there are many supplements on the market which don't provide what they claim. While losing weight, it is critical not to jeopardize your health by using substandard supplements. Detailed content and quality information on the LEAN 51 products can be provided. Be assured that you are taking the very best. Don't miss a dose. Your health, your energy, and your life are moving in a positive direction.

Each step moves you closer to your optimal health and lean weight.

7. Drink 80 oz. of Non-Caloric Beverages Daily

We've all heard the mantra to drink 80-oz. of water daily while losing weight. I agree, with one simple change. Drink 80-oz. of water and a couple of zero calorie beverages a day if you prefer. I believe that water is the best fluid for our bodies, but we have been programmed for taste. If we deprive ourselves of pleasurable tastes, it is harder to stay with a program long enough to lose weight.

There are many flavored and dietary beverages available for consumption. Coffee, tea, diet sodas, flavored waters, and artificially sweetened drinks can be used with the above limitation. It is best to limit the intake of caffeine and artificially sweetened drinks, since some studies suggest these may stimulate hunger. Keeping your body well-hydrated allows the fat-burning machinery to run at top speed. We burn fat better when we are well-hydrated.

Be sure to track your fluid intake on the LEAN 51 Tracker Form.

8. Check Your Attitude

Every day we are confronted with challenges and negativity. If we allow ourselves to focus on the negative it will decrease our ability to lose weight. Working to remain positive and focused on our wonderful future is a choice. It takes effort. Each day, take a little time to think about the good things going on in your life and be grateful for them. Living with an attitude of gratitude will assist you in staying positive. Losing weight and becoming healthy can have its own obstacles. When these frustrations occur, make a solid attempt to refocus on the positive actions you are taking and the successes you have had. Not only are you working on a healthy body, but you are developing a healthy and positive mind.

9. Increase Activity

In my 20 years of practicing medicine, I have known many people who go to the gym, work-out religiously and never lose any weight. In fact, many women stop exercising on a weight loss program because they gain weight. We all know that exercise is important for health and fitness. Most people who are overweight are also in poor physical condition. The last thing they want to do is go on a diet and also have sore muscles every day for 2-3 weeks. The LEAN 51 Program promotes activity in a modest form to begin with. We advise wearing a step tracker every day.

Track the number of steps you take. If you are sedentary and out of shape physically; start slowly and record the number of steps taken each day at your usual activity level. Then we can set goals to help you achieve greater movement over a gradual time frame. A sample chart is shown to give you an idea of how to slowly increase your level of walking. There are no strenuous exercises or training protocols on the LEAN 51 Program. We incorporate healthful walking at your own pace to increase your caloric expenditure.

As you lose the weight, you will gain a tremendous amount of energy. You will naturally increase the number of steps you take each day. Understand that motion creates emotion. As you increase your body's motion, you enhance your positive emotions. Not only will you look great, you will feel great! There is no better way to live long than to feel great while you do it.

10. Partner With Your Coach – Stay in Touch

The LEAN 51 Program provides you with a coach. This is one of the most important parts of your program. Trying to lose weight on our own is difficult and lonely. Having a coach to hold you accountable and to work with you as you move through the program will make the weight loss journey much easier. Your coach understands the LEAN 51 eating plan and will be there to guide you, encourage you, and push you toward your goals.

Your coach and you will decide the best way and times to stay in touch. Emails and in office visits are the best ways to work together. You will develop a special relationship with your coach and can work through any difficulties as well as enjoy your successes together.

When you talk to your coach be sure to have any questions or concerns written down so your time together will be very productive. Also, remember that your coach is not a psychologist, so don't expect therapy sessions. Your communications should focus on the LEAN 51 plan, weight loss, exercise, supplements, the 10 Step Program, information, and celebration.

Your coach is your partner and is provided to you without additional charge. Now, where else can you find a deal like that!

The Goal and the Soul

Every day during the LEAN 51 Program, you will be writing and rewriting your goals. You will also record your thoughts and your feelings as you go through the LEAN 51 Plan. The "Goal" writing portion is self-explanatory. The "Soul" portion is expressing your inner most thoughts and feelings as you experience the changes that are occurring to you as you move through the plan.

I realize that your first reaction to being asked to do this each day is that it is redundant. I assure you that there is a good reason for the repetitive nature of this exercise. Just as you build strong muscles through the repetitive activity of lifting weights, you will build strong goal setting and effective thought changing skills as you write on a daily basis. This activity should only take a few minutes each day.

Women will have no problem with this task, as they are very good at putting their thoughts on paper. Most men, including myself, have difficulty writing our thoughts and feelings down on paper. The best thing to do is to stop thinking about what you have to do and just do the exercise. After a few days you will feel different about the process. You will develop a greater understanding of what it is you are trying to accomplish and how you feel about the fat burning and weight loss process.

Repetition is the mother of habit. You are creating new habits and writing your goals each day which will firmly engrain them in your mind. Your goals may shift or even change a bit as you write them over and over. That's great. You will ultimately define what you want your life to be like as you become more specific with the goals over time. As for the "Soul" writing, you will gain insight into why you have misused food in the past and why it has been so difficult to change your ways. Just so you know the people who have lost the most weight and kept it off over time on the LEAN 51 Program have been the ones that have done their daily writing. Do this for the first 30 days, and if you experience the benefits that I believe you will, continue the process until you reach your lean weight, and for life.

A Lesson About Protein Before Starting

The LEAN 51 Program is a balanced eating program. You will eat a healthful amount of protein, a reduced amount of carbohydrates, and a controlled amount of fat while getting lean. To initiate the process of Lipolysis or fat breakdown, you will eat a higher level of protein than you have been used to before starting the program. By doing this, your body will slowly convert the protein you eat into glucose to use as fuel. Because this occurs slowly and your body requires more fuel than provided by this menu, your fat stores will begin to be used as a source of daily energy.

As these fat stores are burned to provide you with energy, you will notice both weight loss and size reduction. Lean protein and the specially formulated protein snack-meals will be your main source of food during the program. You will receive your carbohydrates and fats from the healthy meal on the plan and from the snack-meals.

Protein is made up of amino acids. The amino acids are converted into glucose in a process that requires our body to expend energy. This energy expenditure is also an important part of the weight loss process. As you cycle through LEAN 51, you will feel less hungry and have greater energy. Be sure to eat lean proteins with your meal. Some are listed on the following page. Good luck as you begin to move quickly toward health.

Picking Proteins

Since you need to eat a protein at each meal, you need some variety to help from getting into the boredom rut. High quality proteins at a reasonable cost can be found on the following list.

- Ground beef, 85% lean or better
- Beef, top round
- Cheese, cheddar, low-fat if possible
- Cottage cheese, fat free
- Chicken breast, skinless
- Egg substitute
- Sliced lean ham
- Canadian bacon
- Low-fat cold cuts (98% fat free)
- Milk, skim or <1%
- Protein powders for shakes
- Protein cereals
- White fish, i.e. cod, tilapia, scrod, lake, or ocean perch
- Salmon
- Tuna, white in water
- Turkey, white
- Ground turkey
- Turkey breast or tenderloins
- Lean pork, trim all fat
- Tofu, low fat
- String cheese, mozzarella
- Soybeans
- Soy Milk
- Non-fat yogurt
- Greek yogurt
- Whole egg

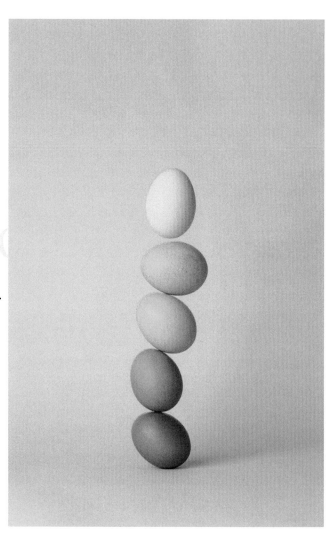

The LEAN 51 Program

Quick Start Guide

KEY POINTS:

- QUICK WEIGHT LOSS: Average weight loss is up to 15 pounds a month
- GREAT TASTE: Portion Controlled Snack-meals are extremely satisfying
- SIMPLE PLAN: Eat every 2 ½ - 3 hours
- '51': 5 Snack-meals a day; 1 Healthy (Lean and Green) meal a day
- NO HUNGER: Eating every 2 ½-3 hours eliminates cravings and hunger
- SUPPORT: Physician and Health Coach support by email
- COST: Lower cost than other programs, and less than or equal to your current food costs per month

Healthy Meal Options

Protein: 4-6 oz. servings
Grilled, baked, broiled, or poached – not fried.

Fish	Chicken	Egg Whites	98% Lean Cold Cuts
Shellfish	Lean Beef	Egg Beaters	Tuna
Game Meats	Lamb	Veggie Burgers	Fat Free Cheese
Turkey	Lean Pork Cuts	Tofu	Low Fat Cottage Cheese

Vegetables: 2 servings (up to 2 cups total)

Celery	Cabbage	Broccoli	Carrots
Cucumber	Mushrooms	Asparagus	Scallions
Lettuce	Peppers	Tomatoes	Onions
Spinach	Radishes	Okra	Squash
Greens	Sprouts	Turnips	Kale
Cauliflower	Eggplant	Green beans	Mixed Veggies/Salad

Condiments: Small amounts of mustard, ketchup, dill pickle, and most herbal and natural seasonings may be used.

Healthy Fats: 2 Tablespoons of regular or low-carb dressing
1 Teaspoon of margarine
1 Tablespoon of Olive Oil

Beverages: Drink 80 oz. of water plus limited zero calorie liquids

1
Healthy Meal
4-6 oz. Lean Protein
2 Vegetable Servings
*Typically lunch or dinner.

5
Snack Meals
Choose From:
Portion Controlled Protein Bars, Shakes, Puddings, Soups, Crunch Bars, Fruit Drinks, and many more available Snack Meals.

Eat one of your 6 meals every 2 ½ - 3 hours

"I have learned to use the word impossible with the greatest of caution"

~Wernher von Braun

DAY 1
Initiation – Convert to Burning Fat

Lesson:

Today you start toward your goal weight. During day one, you will begin to convert your body to a fat burning engine. You will eat more protein today than usual. This allows the body to conserve muscle and switch over to the process of breaking down fat tissue. This switch typically takes 1-3 days. You are now on your way! Be sure to eat every 3 hours and don't miss any snack-meals. You will not eat fruits, grains, or foods typically having high carbohydrates in them. You will get enough carbohydrates, which are a part of the snack-meals and healthy meal vegetables on the plan.

LEAN 51 is not intended to eliminate carbohydrates. Your intake of carbohydrates will be in the 75-100 gram range each day. You should not eat unlimited amounts of protein either. Some dietary fads recommend eating all of the protein you can. These are excess calories you don't need or utilize. A serving of protein at your one healthy lean meal should be 4-6 oz. The snack-meals are portion controlled. If you are having any difficulty with hunger in the first 3 days, eat an additional snack-meal serving. These snack-meals should get you through the day without experiencing hunger, cravings or weakness. You are eating every 2 ½-3 hours. Send us an e-mail this week so we can track your initial response and progress as you turn on your fat burning machinery.

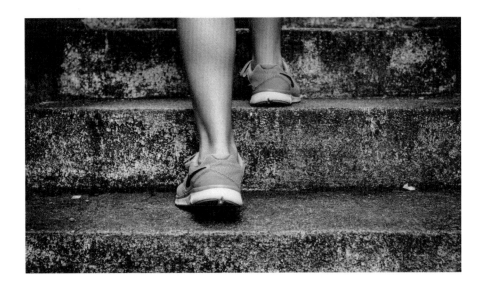

LEAN 51   DAILY TRACKER

Check off each item throughout the day to keep track of food, vitamins, water, and exercise.

Day # _____   Weight _____   Vitamin Pack _____

Your Daily Dietary Plan

Snack-Meal #1 _____   (Eat this first meal within 1 hour of arising)

Snack-Meal #2 _____

Snack-Meal #3 _____   **Daily Fluid intake**

Snack-Meal #4 _____   each box equals 8oz.

Snack-Meal #5 _____

Healthy Lean Meal   Protein   _____

2 Vegetables _____   Step Reading:_____

"Journaling is like whispering to one's self and listening at the same time."

~ Mina Murray

THE GOAL AND THE SOUL

Daily Goals

Write your goals in the space provided. These are your weight loss goals, your change-in-eating goals, your fitness and exercise goals and any other goals you want to achieve over time. Writing and re-writing goals daily is very powerful.

_____

_____

_____

_____

_____

_____

_____

Daily Soul
(Your Journal)

Write your feelings, thoughts and ideas below. These should include things you learned today, things you are excited about today, and things that you are grateful for today. Include any other details of the day you believe are important. This is your private workbook. Be honest with yourself. How do you really feel? Get it out of your head and on paper!

_____

_____

_____

_____

_____

_____

_____

What's Your Story
(Tasks and Victories)

_____

_____

_____

_____

_____

_____

_____

_____

_____

_____

Act as if it were impossible to fail."

~ Dorothea Brande

DAY 2
FAT BURNING DEVELOPING

Lesson:

Lesson: On Day 1 or Day 2, 70% of people start to burn fat. Fat is turned into ketone bodies. Ketones are fuel for the body and brain, which are derived from fat (adipose) tissue. Some people test their urine for the presence of ketones to determine fat breakdown, but this is not necessary. Staying on the LEAN 51 plan will break down fat. You're off to a great start! Our bodies can only burn two fuels. One is glucose, which is preferred by our body. The other is ketones. The LEAN 51 Program will "flip the switch" to using ketones for fuel, which are the breakdown product of fat. You will literally turn those fat stores in your body into high energy fuel.

The ketones also protect you from cravings and give you a sense of energy, decreased hunger, and mental well-being. When you awaken in the morning you will begin to feel more energy. These ketones, that are your fuel source from fat, are in no way harmful to your body. Some people confuse the medical condition of ketoacidosis in Type I diabetes with ketosis of fat breakdown. Though the ketones are the same, the extremely high ketone level of ketoacidosis is unique to uncontrolled Type I diabetics. If you are not a Type I diabetic, then the production of ketones for fuel is a normal process of eliminating fat from the body by using it as fuel. Oh, by the way, congratulations on getting started. You are a winner!

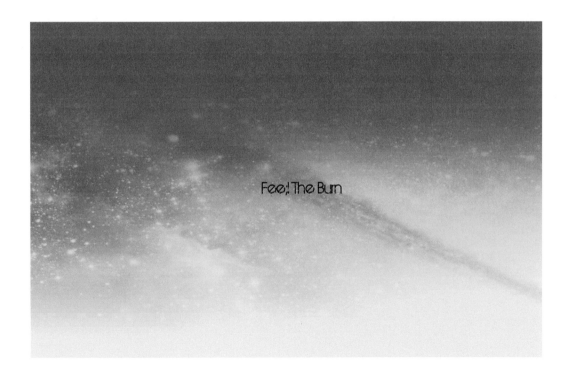
Feel The Burn

LEAN 51 DAILY TRACKER

Check off each item throughout the day to keep track of food, vitamins, water, and exercise.

Day # _____   Weight _____   Vitamin Pack _____

Your Daily Dietary Plan

Snack-Meal #1 _____   (Eat this first meal within 1 hour of arising)

Snack-Meal #2 _____

Snack-Meal #3 _____   **Daily Fluid intake**
each box equals 8oz.

Snack-Meal #4 _____

Snack-Meal #5 _____

Healthy Lean Meal   Protein   _____

2 Vegetables _____   Step Reading:_____

"Journaling is like whispering to one's self and listening at the same time."

~ Mina Murray

THE GOAL AND THE SOUL

Daily Goals

Write your goals in the space provided. These are your weight loss goals, your change-in-eating goals, your fitness and exercise goals and any other goals you want to achieve over time. Writing and re-writing goals daily is very powerful.

_____

_____

_____

_____

_____

_____

_____

Daily Soul
(Your Journal)

Write your feelings, thoughts and ideas below. These should include things you learned today, things you are excited about today, and things that you are grateful for today. Include any other details of the day you believe are important. This is your private workbook. Be honest with yourself. How do you really feel? Get it out of your head and on paper!

_____

_____

_____

_____

_____

_____

<u>What's Your Story</u>
(Tasks and Victories)

_____

_____

_____

_____

_____

_____

_____

_____

_____

_____

_____

_____

"We can accomplish almost anything within our ability if we but think that we can."

~ George Matthew Adams

Day 3

Fat Reduction Well Underway: Lipolysis (Converting Fat to Fuel)

Lesson

You've now jump-started the fat loss process. Today you will continue to eat every 3 hours with your snack-meals and your Healthy Lean Meal. You will eat approximately 75-100 grams of carbohydrates a day. You are now on an "enhanced protein, reduced carbohydrate, controlled fat dietary regimen. This is eating healthy. You are burning more calories than you are taking in. Your body will soon match your mindset. Review your goals now. Today you are one step closer to them!

Many people ask me what the "special ingredient" or "magic" of the LEAN 51 Program is. This is probably because of all the marketing and advertising for items like "fat burners", "metabolism boosters", and "special diet formulas" to melt away fat. Unfortunately, these don't exist. If they did, I would be prescribing them to patients in my practice. I tell patients that if these claims were true, every doctor in America would be using them to help their patients. I also tell them that if these items worked, 80% of Americans would not be overweight.

The magic behind the LEAN 51 Program is that it provides sound nutrition at the appropriate time of the day in the appropriate quantities to allow your own body's natural process to burn up the stored fat and protect the calorie burning muscle tissue. This change in fat/muscle ratio increases your metabolic rate and helps sustain long-term weight loss.

There is one magical thing about the LEAN 51 Program. It's the team members like you that contribute back to others with your experience that makes this so special. It is an honor to have you as a partner.

Our vision is to assist people to Live Lean, Living Long, and Live Life to the Fullest.

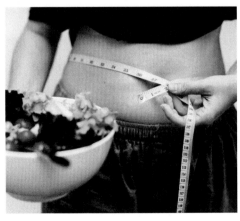

LEAN 51   DAILY TRACKER

Check off each item throughout the day to keep track of food, vitamins, water, and exercise.

Day # _____   Weight _____   Vitamin Pack _____

Your Daily Dietary Plan

Snack-Meal #1 _____   (Eat this first meal within 1 hour of arising)

Snack-Meal #2 _____

Snack-Meal #3 _____

Snack-Meal #4 _____

Snack-Meal #5 _____

Daily Fluid intake
each box equals 8oz.

Healthy Lean Meal   Protein   _____

2 Vegetables _____   Step Reading:_____

"Journaling is like whispering to one's self and listening at the same time."

~ Mina Murray

THE GOAL AND THE SOUL

Daily Goals

Write your goals in the space provided. These are your weight loss goals, your change-in-eating goals, your fitness and exercise goals and any other goals you want to achieve over time. Writing and re-writing goals daily is very powerful.

_____

_____

_____

_____

_____

_____

Daily Soul
(Your Journal)

Write your feelings, thoughts and ideas below. These should include things you learned today, things you are excited about today, and things that you are grateful for today. Include any other details of the day you believe are important. This is your private workbook. Be honest with yourself. How do you really feel? Get it out of your head and on paper!

_____

_____

_____

_____

_____

_____

What's Your Story
(Tasks and Victories)

_____

_____

_____

_____

_____

_____

_____

_____

_____

_____

Always bear in mind that your own resolution to success is more important than any other one thing."

~ Abraham Lincoln

DAY 4
Fat Burning Engine Turned On

Lesson:

On Day 4 of the LEAN 51 Program, almost everyone feels less hungry and more energetic. If you do not, let us know. This eating pattern is a change from your past eating behaviors and some people experience some "carbohydrate withdrawal." It's only an emotional feeling, but can make you feel deprived. Remember, you are getting plenty of food, more variety and you are losing fat and excess weight. I am proud of you!

The most difficult part of any project is getting started. You have already completed that difficult task. It's truly amazing how many people will invest in a project or program and never even cross the starting line. You are not that type of person. You are already on Day 4. You are committed to your vision of a lean, healthful lifestyle.

There is nothing that can stop you from achieving that goal. Fill in your daily tracker and write down your thoughts. Most people have a strong sense of excitement and a boost of self-energy and confidence today. Let us know your thoughts. Rest well tonight. Review your vision and your goals. Your fat-burning engine is now running efficiently.

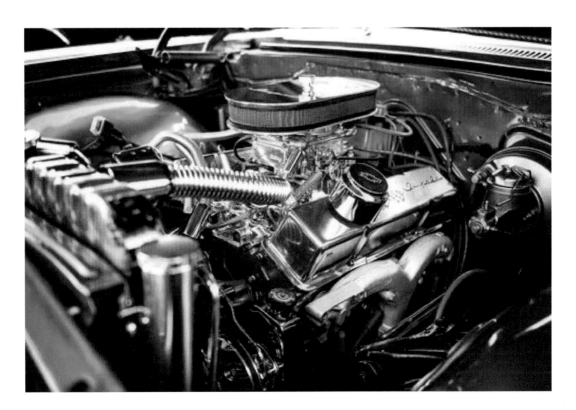

LEAN 51   DAILY TRACKER

Check off each item throughout the day to keep track of food, vitamins, water, and exercise.

Day # _____   Weight _____   Vitamin Pack _____

Your Daily Dietary Plan

Snack-Meal #1 _____   (Eat this first meal within 1 hour of arising)

Snack-Meal #2 _____

Snack-Meal #3 _____   **Daily Fluid intake**
                                         each box equals 8oz.
Snack-Meal #4 _____

Snack-Meal #5 _____

Healthy Lean Meal   Protein   _____

               2 Vegetables _____   Step Reading:_____

"Journaling is like whispering to one's self and listening at the same time."

~ Mina Murray

THE GOAL AND THE SOUL

Daily Goals

Write your goals in the space provided. These are your weight loss goals, your change-in-eating goals, your fitness and exercise goals and any other goals you want to achieve over time. Writing and re-writing goals daily is very powerful.

_____

_____

_____

_____

_____

_____

Daily Soul
(Your Journal)

Write your feelings, thoughts and ideas below. These should include things you learned today, things you are excited about today, and things that you are grateful for today. Include any other details of the day you believe are important. This is your private workbook. Be honest with yourself. How do you really feel? Get it out of your head and on paper!

_____

_____

_____

_____

_____

_____

_____

What's Your Story
(Tasks and Victories)

_____

_____

_____

_____

_____

_____

_____

_____

_____

"It is the greatest shot of adrenaline to be doing what you've wanted to do so badly. You almost feel like you could fly without the plane."

~ Charles Lindbergh

DAY 5
Fat Reduction Continues 24/7

Lesson:

When you "dieted" before, you deprived yourself of food. You got your mind ready to eliminate foods and get by on as little as possible. You didn't want to do it, but felt no other options were available. After 4-5 days, you were miserable. On the LEAN 51 Plan, you are eating every three hours. The snack-meals are chewy and tasty and you wonder how you will eat all of this food. Each day you are developing the habit of healthy eating. No more starvation! No more deprivation!

If deprivation and dieting methods of the past worked, you would already be living at your ideal body weight. You know they don't. It is sometimes difficult to change how we feel about losing weight. I know that it is hard to believe that eating more often would promote rapid fat loss. Fortunately, you are already seeing the benefits of the LEAN 51 Plan. If you're like most people, by now you are noticing changes. These changes come from improved nutrition, elimination of excess fluids and waste, ketosis, and the elimination of missed meals and past overeating habits.

These changes are promoting a dramatic improvement in your body, your mind, and your commitment. You are burning fat while you're working, playing, walking, and even while you sleep. The fluffy, floppy, fat tissue is slowly shrinking away uncovering the lean, strong, fit person underneath it. You are the artist sculpting the new you. Be excited!

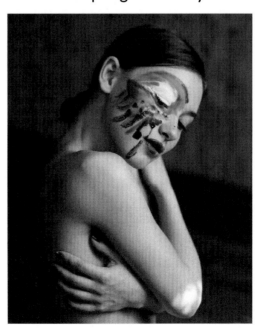

LEAN 51   DAILY TRACKER

Check off each item throughout the day to keep track of food, vitamins, water, and exercise.

Day # _____   Weight _____   Vitamin Pack _____

Your Daily Dietary Plan

Snack-Meal #1 _____   (Eat this first meal within 1 hour of arising)

Snack-Meal #2 _____

Daily Fluid intake

Snack-Meal #3 _____   each box equals 8oz.

Snack-Meal #4 _____

Snack-Meal #5 _____

Healthy Lean Meal   Protein   _____

2 Vegetables _____   Step Reading:_____

"Journaling is like whispering to one's self and listening at the same time."

~ Mina Murray

THE GOAL AND THE SOUL

Daily Goals

Write your goals in the space provided. These are your weight loss goals, your change-in-eating goals, your fitness and exercise goals and any other goals you want to achieve over time. Writing and re-writing goals daily is very powerful.

_____

_____

_____

_____

_____

_____

_____

Daily Soul
(Your Journal)

Write your feelings, thoughts and ideas below. These should include things you learned today, things you are excited about today, and things that you are grateful for today. Include any other details of the day you believe are important. This is your private workbook. Be honest with yourself. How do you really feel? Get it out of your head and on paper!

_____

_____

_____

_____

_____

_____

<u>What's Your Story</u>
(Tasks and Victories)

_____

_____

_____

_____

_____

_____

_____

_____

_____

_____

_____

"Keep your promises to yourself."

~ David Harold Fink

DAY 6
Fat Burning is Fun

Lesson:

Where are those cravings you used to have on diets? Because you are giving your body fuel as it needs it, you are not getting hungry. Be sure to eat your snack-meals. If you do sense hunger, have an additional snack-meal. You are eating 6 times a day. There is no space in your day for cravings to attack. You are now "snacking" your way to health. Your body is getting the nutrients it needs at the right time to provide you with all the energy you require. Keep snacking, keep losing!

One of the greatest benefits for me is seeing the smiles on patient's faces during the early stages of the program. You probably have one on your face right now. I believe it comes from the knowledge that you really are in control of your future. You have been given the awesome gift of choice and you are using it right now to live a healthier way.

Feeling in control is powerful. Knowing that those days of frustration and feeling helpless due to your excess weight are over and it lifts your spirit to a new level. I believe you are here to do wonderful things with your life. In order to do that, you must do wonderful things for your life. Getting lean, getting fit, and developing life-prolonging habits will allow you to be the best at the rest of your life's endeavors.

So smile big – Be happy and enjoy the journey you are taking. Live Lean, Live Long, Live Life to the Fullest!!

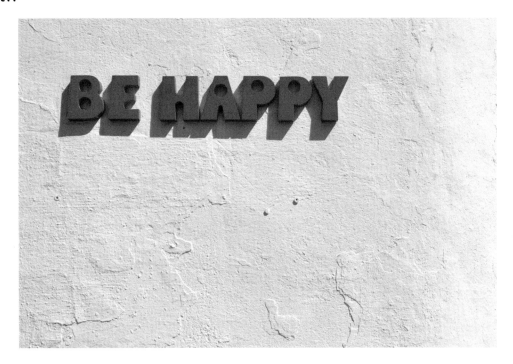

LEAN 51   DAILY TRACKER

Check off each item throughout the day to keep track of food, vitamins, water, and exercise.

Day # _____   Weight _____   Vitamin Pack _____

Your Daily Dietary Plan

Snack-Meal #1 _____   (Eat this first meal within 1 hour of arising)

Snack-Meal #2 _____

Snack-Meal #3 _____

Daily Fluid intake
each box equals 8oz.

Snack-Meal #4 _____

Snack-Meal #5 _____

Healthy Lean Meal   Protein   _____

2 Vegetables _____   Step Reading:_____

"Journaling is like whispering to one's self and listening at the same time."

~ Mina Murray

THE GOAL AND THE SOUL

Daily Goals

Write your goals in the space provided. These are your weight loss goals, your change-in-eating goals, your fitness and exercise goals and any other goals you want to achieve over time. Writing and re-writing goals daily is very powerful.

_____

_____

_____

_____

_____

_____

_____

Daily Soul
(Your Journal)

Write your feelings, thoughts and ideas below. These should include things you learned today, things you are excited about today, and things that you are grateful for today. Include any other details of the day you believe are important. This is your private workbook. Be honest with yourself. How do you really feel? Get it out of your head and on paper!

_____

_____

_____

_____

_____

What's Your Story
(Tasks and Victories)

"Life is the sum of all your choices."

~ Albert Carmus

DAY 7
Check Your Progress – Great Job!

Lesson:

You have been weighing yourself each day. You have been tracking your steps, your fluid intake, your food intake, and other critical measurements. After 1 week, you should see a change in your weight. If you've lost 2-5 pounds, that's great. Many will have lost more. Some of this loss above 2-5 pounds is water and internal waste elimination. You say "who cares?', "weight loss is weight loss and I'm excited." It's very important to continue to use your check-off tracker each day. Let us know how much you've lost in week 1 by e-mail. We are excited for you!

It's easy to get excited with the progress you have made. Keep focused on the day to day changes you are making. Each simple change is being etched in your mind. Repetition of these new daily habits will become a permanent part of your life. You are becoming very good at preparing your meals, keeping the snack-meals with you and wearing your step tracker. Don't let the simplicity of this program allow you to start leaving out any of the steps.

The magic of life long weight control lies in the daily pattern you are currently establishing. You have most likely seen this pattern in people you know who have always been lean. They eat when they are hungry and don't eat when they are not. They take those few extra steps everywhere they go and don't even think about it. They eat vegetables with each meal and keep their portions under control. From this point on, you are one of them. You are already lean in your mind. Your body is following close behind. Keep it simple, be repetitive, and learn the LEAN 51 way.

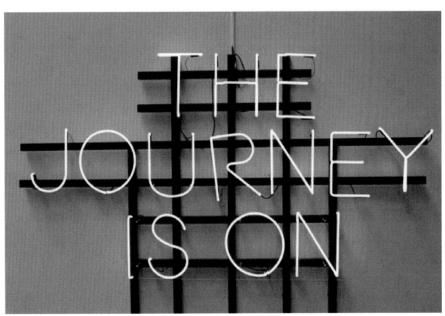

LEAN 51   DAILY TRACKER

Check off each item throughout the day to keep track of food, vitamins, water, and exercise.

Day # _____   Weight _____   Vitamin Pack _____

Your Daily Dietary Plan

Snack-Meal #1 _____   (Eat this first meal within 1 hour of arising)

Snack-Meal #2 _____

Snack-Meal #3 _____   **Daily Fluid intake**

Snack-Meal #4 _____   each box equals 8oz.

Snack-Meal #5 _____

Healthy Lean Meal   Protein   _____

2 Vegetables _____   Step Reading:_____

"Journaling is like whispering to one's self and listening at the same time."

~ Mina Murray

THE GOAL AND THE SOUL

Daily Goals

Write your goals in the space provided. These are your weight loss goals, your change-in-eating goals, your fitness and exercise goals and any other goals you want to achieve over time. Writing and re-writing goals daily is very powerful.

_____

_____

_____

_____

_____

_____

_____

Daily Soul
(Your Journal)

Write your feelings, thoughts and ideas below. These should include things you learned today, things you are excited about today, and things that you are grateful for today. Include any other details of the day you believe are important. This is your private workbook. Be honest with yourself. How do you really feel? Get it out of your head and on paper!

_____

_____

_____

_____

_____

What's Your Story
(Tasks and Victories)

"It's never too later - in fiction or in life - to revise."

~ Nancy Thayer

Day 8
Thinking a New Way

Lesson:

You are not a fat person! You are a normal person with too much fat on your body. Unfortunately, we label ourselves as we see ourselves. Today it's time to change your thinking. You must see yourself in your own mind as a lean, fit, healthy person. You must change your thinking. You must picture yourself each day at your optimum weight. Visualize yourself in new clothes that fit well. See yourself in your body the way it was meant to be. You are living a healthy and vibrant life. You are healthy! Say to yourself each day – "I'm lean, I'm fit, and I'm strong!"

When you truly know that you are eating right and see yourself as a fit and trim individual, you are on your way to a lifetime of health and vitality. Many scholars and philosophers have discovered that when we believe in something so much and know that it's a part of who we are, then our innermost mind and thought will lead us to our desire. I know that your desire is to be lean and healthy. Convincing yourself that you are worthy of that goal will be the most difficult part of the journey. I think you are worthy of your goal.

In your journal today, write down the phrase: "I'm lean, I'm fit, and I'm strong!" Say it to yourself several times a day. I like to say it out loud when I'm exercising. It makes a nice rhythmic sound as I match it to my footsteps. If this all sounds new or even silly to you, that's OK. Just try it. Remember, thinking and doing what you've always done won't get you where you want to be. It's time to think in a new way. Think Lean, Think Fit, Think Strong!

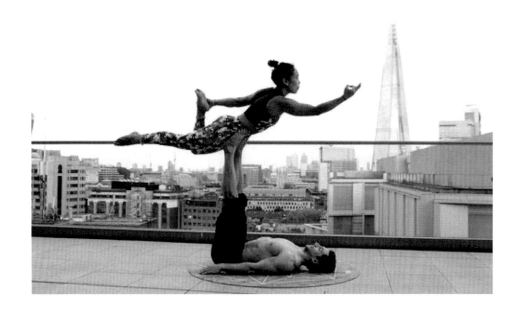

LEAN 51   DAILY TRACKER

Check off each item throughout the day to keep track of food, vitamins, water, and exercise.

Day # _____   Weight _____   Vitamin Pack _____

Your Daily Dietary Plan

Snack-Meal #1 _____   (Eat this first meal within 1 hour of arising)

Snack-Meal #2 _____

Snack-Meal #3 _____   **Daily Fluid intake**

each box equals 8oz.

Snack-Meal #4 _____

Snack-Meal #5 _____

Healthy Lean Meal   Protein   _____

2 Vegetables _____   Step Reading:_____

"Journaling is like whispering to one's self and listening at the same time."

~ Mina Murray

THE GOAL AND THE SOUL

Daily Goals

Write your goals in the space provided. These are your weight loss goals, your change-in-eating goals, your fitness and exercise goals and any other goals you want to achieve over time. Writing and re-writing goals daily is very powerful.

_____

_____

_____

_____

_____

_____

Daily Soul
(Your Journal)

Write your feelings, thoughts and ideas below. These should include things you learned today, things you are excited about today, and things that you are grateful for today. Include any other details of the day you believe are important. This is your private workbook. Be honest with yourself. How do you really feel? Get it out of your head and on paper!

_____

_____

_____

_____

_____

_____

<u>What's Your Story</u>
(Tasks and Victories)

_____

_____

_____

_____

_____

_____

_____

_____

_____

_____

"To remain young one must change."

~ Alexander Chase

DAY 9
The Magic of Fluids

Lesson:

Our bodies are over 70% water. Water is critical to our health and wellbeing. Though clean, well-filtered water is a must, you can get your daily fluid requirements from many sources. On the LEAN 51 Program, you can drink any non-caloric beverage with limitation. Non-calorie-flavored waters are a big hit and are available at most grocers and large discount stores. Coffee, tea, and diet soft drinks are allowed. Newer studies show that drinking fluids with artificial sweeteners may still stimulate our appetite. Keep the number of "diet" drinks to 1 or 2 daily. Limit your daily caffeine, as it sometimes contributes to increased appetite. So, here's to your health – Drink up!

Keeping your body well-hydrated will keep the internal machinery running smoothly. The waste products of fat burning will be rinsed from your system by these fluids. Your cells and your organs will be bathed in life-promoting water. The energy rich food that you now eat will supply nutrients to your body through your enhanced blood flow. When I draw blood samples from patients with too much fat in their body and blood, what I see is startling. We spin the blood in our lab to separate the cells from the plasma.

In these over-fat patients, the plasma is not clear as it should be. It looks like thick yellowed milk and there is a layer of fat that collects between the red cells and the plasma that looks like butter. This layer consists of triglycerides and other fats. On the LEAN 51 Program, you have already begun to cleanse yourself of these unneeded and unwanted substances. You can be assured that your body is ridding itself of these toxins. Remember, by living this new way, you will be living longer. So today, drink to your good health –at least 80-ounces.

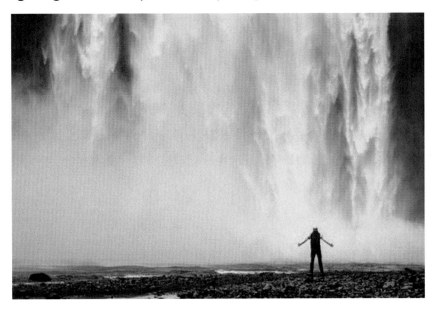

LEAN 51   DAILY TRACKER

Check off each item throughout the day to keep track of food, vitamins, water, and exercise.

Day # _____   Weight _____   Vitamin Pack _____

Your Daily Dietary Plan

Snack-Meal #1 _____   (Eat this first meal within 1 hour of arising)

Snack-Meal #2 _____

Snack-Meal #3 _____   ## Daily Fluid intake
each box equals 8oz.

Snack-Meal #4 _____

Snack-Meal #5 _____

Healthy Lean Meal   Protein   _____

2 Vegetables _____   Step Reading:_____

"Journaling is like whispering to one's self and listening at the same time."

~ Mina Murray

THE GOAL AND THE SOUL

Daily Goals

Write your goals in the space provided. These are your weight loss goals, your change-in-eating goals, your fitness and exercise goals and any other goals you want to achieve over time. Writing and re-writing goals daily is very powerful.

_____

_____

_____

_____

_____

_____

Daily Soul
(Your Journal)

Write your feelings, thoughts and ideas below. These should include things you learned today, things you are excited about today, and things that you are grateful for today. Include any other details of the day you believe are important. This is your private workbook. Be honest with yourself. How do you really feel? Get it out of your head and on paper!

_____

_____

_____

_____

_____

What's Your Story
(Tasks and Victories)

"Where the willingness is great, the difficulties cannot be great."

~ Niccolo Machiavelli

DAY 10
The Menu is Magical

Lesson:

Follow the menu closely. In the past, it was easy to get to the end of your day and not even recall what you had to eat as you went from waking to bedtime. Now that you are on the LEAN 51 plan, you must follow the recommended menu as part of the training. Eventually, your body and mind will incorporate this new eating pattern into habit. You have chosen to become leaner and eating foods or snacks not on the program will delay your progress and frustrate you. You will not be hungry on the LEAN 51 plan and you will feel so good about yourself when you are disciplined with it. Remember, nothing tastes as good as thin feels.

There are many diets on the market and I'm sure you've tried them all. Most experts believe that a balanced diet is the best diet. The LEAN 51 menu is formulated to give your body the proper nutrients at the right time. By having protein at least 6 times a day, you will be assured of having a steady blood glucose (sugar) level all day long. The snack-meals will give you some added energy throughout the day and the vegetables in the healthy meal provide fiber and valuable phytochemicals for proper digestion and elimination.

No single component is left out of the LEAN 51 menu as is the case in several popular programs. Our bodies were created to use proteins, carbohydrates, and fats; and, leaving any of these out will adversely affect our health. I sometimes have patients say "I can't eat vegetables." I've yet to find this to be true. You may not like vegetables, but you can find at least 2 or 3 of them that will satisfy you. Stop thinking what you can't do, and focus on what you can do. Eat precisely what is on the menu and you will be pleased with your results and progress. If you feel you have specials needs, please contact us to discuss these.

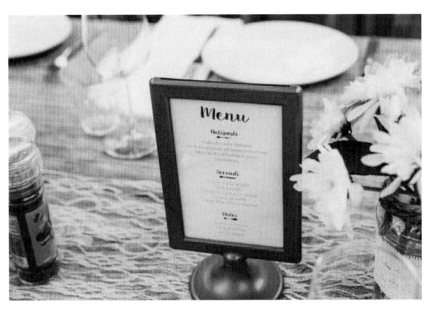

LEAN 51   DAILY TRACKER

Check off each item throughout the day to keep track of food, vitamins, water, and exercise.

Day # _____   Weight _____   Vitamin Pack _____

Your Daily Dietary Plan

Snack-Meal #1 _____   (Eat this first meal within 1 hour of arising)

Snack-Meal #2 _____

Snack-Meal #3 _____   **Daily Fluid intake**
                                            each box equals 8oz.

Snack-Meal #4 _____

Snack-Meal #5 _____

Healthy Lean Meal   Protein   _____

                  2 Vegetables _____   Step Reading:_____

"Journaling is like whispering to one's self and listening at the same time."

~ Mina Murray

THE GOAL AND THE SOUL

Daily Goals

Write your goals in the space provided. These are your weight loss goals, your change-in-eating goals, your fitness and exercise goals and any other goals you want to achieve over time. Writing and re-writing goals daily is very powerful.

_____

_____

_____

_____

_____

_____

_____

Daily Soul
(Your Journal)

Write your feelings, thoughts and ideas below. These should include things you learned today, things you are excited about today, and things that you are grateful for today. Include any other details of the day you believe are important. This is your private workbook. Be honest with yourself. How do you really feel? Get it out of your head and on paper!

_____

_____

_____

_____

_____

_____

_____

What's Your Story
(Tasks and Victories)

_____

_____

_____

_____

_____

_____

_____

_____

_____

_____

"What one has to do usually can be done"

~ Eleanor Rooseelt

DAY 11
Breakfast for Champions

Lesson:

Our American lifestyle is fast-paced and extremely busy. Most of us get out of bed at the last minute. (Gotta get that last minute of shut-eye.) We rush around to get through our morning ritual and race off to work without eating breakfast. Now your body is operating at a deficit in the fuel department. About 9:00 – 10:00 am, you've reached your empty mark and you search the office or workplace for a quick fix.

Ah, the donut or other high-sugar pick-me-up. The problem is eating like this and working a sedentary job "teaches" your body to build fat. You don't need high calories at that time so the extra carbohydrates from the sweets are converted to fat for storage. The solution – Don't skip breakfast. After all, it's on your menu. Have your first meal or snack meal within one hour of waking up.

I like to think of our bodies in the same way I think about my car. I would never try to drive my car without giving it fuel first. If I did, I wouldn't get where I was going. The same holds true for your body. If you don't give it fuel, you won't get where you want to go. Oh sure, you will make it through the day feeling tired and being irritable. That's no way to live. The most common complaint I get in my office is that of fatigue and lethargy. When questioned, almost every person with that complaint doesn't eat first thing in the morning, misses meals, and grabs fast food on the run. They don't exercise and have poor sleep habits.

If you've been one of these people, your life is in the process of changing. Your new eating and exercise habits are already improving your energy levels. So, keep fuel in the tank, eat every meal or snack meal, and you will get where you are going.

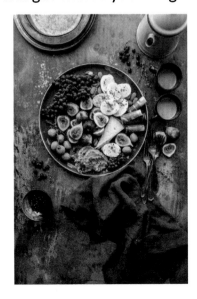

LEAN 51   DAILY TRACKER

Check off each item throughout the day to keep track of food, vitamins, water, and exercise.

Day # _____   Weight _____   Vitamin Pack _____

Your Daily Dietary Plan

Snack-Meal #1 _____   (Eat this first meal within 1 hour of arising)

Snack-Meal #2 _____

Snack-Meal #3 _____

Daily Fluid intake
each box equals 8oz.

Snack-Meal #4 _____

Snack-Meal #5 _____

Healthy Lean Meal   Protein   _____

2 Vegetables _____   Step Reading:_____

"Journaling is like whispering to one's self and listening at the same time."

~ Mina Murray

THE GOAL AND THE SOUL

Daily Goals

Write your goals in the space provided. These are your weight loss goals, your change-in-eating goals, your fitness and exercise goals and any other goals you want to achieve over time. Writing and re-writing goals daily is very powerful.

_____

_____

_____

_____

_____

_____

Daily Soul
(Your Journal)

Write your feelings, thoughts and ideas below. These should include things you learned today, things you are excited about today, and things that you are grateful for today. Include any other details of the day you believe are important. This is your private workbook. Be honest with yourself. How do you really feel? Get it out of your head and on paper!

_____

_____

_____

_____

What's Your Story
(Tasks and Victories)

"The dedicated life is the life worth living."

~ Annie Dillard

DAY 12
The "Craving" Monster

Lesson:

By eating the right foods at the appropriate times, you have eliminated the vast majority of cravings. The protein snack-meals are specifically designed to give your body ample fuel and satisfy your taste. If you experience occasional cravings or hunger pangs, you can have an additional snack-meal. Some larger individuals may require additional snack-meals a day and still lose weight. If you are unsure about any menu adjustments to avoid cravings, send us an e-mail. We'll set you on the right path. Many of our clients have informed us that the snack-meals are the magic of the program. Be sure you fully experience this magic. Enjoy your snack-meals!

Mark S. is a LEAN 51 success story. He has lost 170 pounds since starting the program. He tells me that at the beginning of his weight loss journey, he would eat an extra 1-2 snack-meals a day. This is what it took for him to satisfy the hunger. At his much reduced weight, he eats the recommended number of snack-meals, but doesn't hesitate to have an additional snack-meal if he feels a significant craving. He now has great insight into living a healthier life.

Mark and I want you to reach your goal and become a LEAN 51 success story like so many others have already done. If you've not already found a picture of yourself that disgusts you, find one today. Put it somewhere to motivate you. Mark carries his "before" picture with him. He never wants to go back and keeps the reminder close at hand. Mark has killed his craving monster. Now it's your turn!

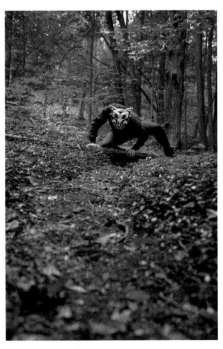

LEAN 51   DAILY TRACKER

Check off each item throughout the day to keep track of food, vitamins, water, and exercise.

Day # _____   Weight _____   Vitamin Pack _____

Your Daily Dietary Plan

Snack-Meal #1 _____   (Eat this first meal within 1 hour of arising)

Snack-Meal #2 _____

Snack-Meal #3 _____   **Daily Fluid intake**

each box equals 8oz.

Snack-Meal #4 _____

Snack-Meal #5 _____

Healthy Lean Meal   Protein   _____

2 Vegetables _____   Step Reading:_____

"Journaling is like whispering to one's self and listening at the same time."

~ Mina Murray

THE GOAL AND THE SOUL

Daily Goals

Write your goals in the space provided. These are your weight loss goals, your change-in-eating goals, your fitness and exercise goals and any other goals you want to achieve over time. Writing and re-writing goals daily is very powerful.

_____

_____

_____

_____

_____

_____

Daily Soul
(Your Journal)

Write your feelings, thoughts and ideas below. These should include things you learned today, things you are excited about today, and things that you are grateful for today. Include any other details of the day you believe are important. This is your private workbook. Be honest with yourself. How do you really feel? Get it out of your head and on paper!

_____

_____

_____

_____

_____

_____

_____

What's Your Story
(Tasks and Victories)

_____

_____

_____

_____

_____

_____

_____

_____

_____

_____

"Yesterday I dared to struggle. Today I dare to win."

~ Bernadette Devlin

DAY 13
You're on the Team

Lesson:

We like to think of our clients as part of our Team – Our LEAN Team. Doing things alone is never as much fun as doing them with friends and family. Ask a friend or family member to be your partner in the LEAN 51 Program. Even if they don't need to lose weight, they will learn a great deal about eating healthier and feeling better.

Touching base with someone each day strengthens our accountability. If you don't have someone to partner with, partner with us. Being part of the team can be motivational and supportive. We find that those who stay in contact with our health coaches lose more weight, lose it faster and keep it off. Our Team is on a mission to Fight Fat and Feel Fantastic. Welcome to the Team!

We are here to be your coaches. We know that it's sometimes lonely when you are trying to lose the excess weight. A team works together to help each other achieve victory. As our team member, you bring your commitment and excitement to us. Others will benefit from your success and you will benefit from theirs'. If you have ideas which promote health and fitness, please let us know. Your input, as a valued team member, is vital to our mission to Live Lean, Live Long, Live Life to the Fullest!

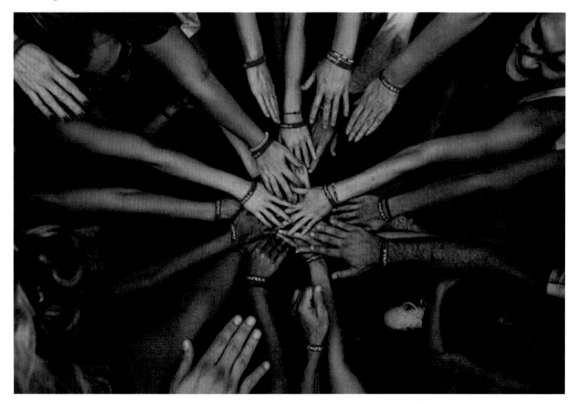

LEAN 51   DAILY TRACKER

Check off each item throughout the day to keep track of food, vitamins, water, and exercise.

Day # _____   Weight _____   Vitamin Pack _____

Your Daily Dietary Plan

Snack-Meal #1 _____   (Eat this first meal within 1 hour of arising)

Snack-Meal #2 _____

Snack-Meal #3 _____   **Daily Fluid intake**
each box equals 8oz.

Snack-Meal #4 _____

Snack-Meal #5 _____

Healthy Lean Meal   Protein   _____

            2 Vegetables _____   Step Reading:_____

"Journaling is like whispering to one's self and listening at the same time."

~ Mina Murray

THE GOAL AND THE SOUL

Daily Goals

Write your goals in the space provided. These are your weight loss goals, your change-in-eating goals, your fitness and exercise goals and any other goals you want to achieve over time. Writing and re-writing goals daily is very powerful.

_____

_____

_____

_____

_____

_____

Daily Soul
(Your Journal)

Write your feelings, thoughts and ideas below. These should include things you learned today, things you are excited about today, and things that you are grateful for today. Include any other details of the day you believe are important. This is your private workbook. Be honest with yourself. How do you really feel? Get it out of your head and on paper!

_____

_____

_____

_____

_____

<u>What's Your Story</u>
(Tasks and Victories)

_____

_____

_____

_____

_____

_____

_____

_____

_____

_____

"One of the biggest factors is the courage to undertake something."

~ James A. Worsham

DAY 14
Scaling Down

Lesson:

When patients come to my office we weigh them at each visit. One problem is we have a separate scale in each exam room. When patients weigh on different scales they see variation in their weight and weight loss. This will happen to you if your use multiple scales to weigh on. To solve this problem, use the same scale throughout your program to get a real measurement of your achievement. Pick a scale at home, at the gym, or at your doctor's office and weigh on it every time. Make sure it is correctly calibrated. By doing this you will avoid frustration that's not your fault. Just a tip – hope it helps.

Several of our more detailed-oriented members have a large sheet of graph paper on the wall at home near their scales. There are also blue tooth enabled scales that send data to your smartphone or computer. They plot their daily weights and can see the drop in pounds over time. This adds to their positive feelings about the great results. I used a computer-tracking program, which plotted out my daily weights as I moved through the program. When I reached my goal, I was amazed at the path of the graph.

While you don't have to do this, try to find small ways to remind yourself daily that you are winning ground every day. When you have reached your goal weight and are healthy, we'll pass on the things that elped you to other team members. Remember, the scale is not your enemy. It is just a tool. Use it daily. It will soon become your friend.

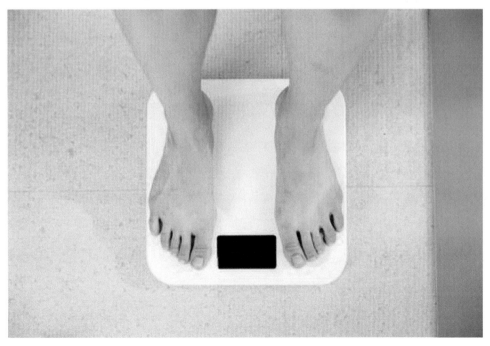

LEAN 51   DAILY TRACKER

Check off each item throughout the day to keep track of food, vitamins, water, and exercise.

Day # _____   Weight _____   Vitamin Pack _____

Your Daily Dietary Plan

Snack-Meal #1 _____   (Eat this first meal within 1 hour of arising)

Snack-Meal #2 _____

Snack-Meal #3 _____

Daily Fluid intake

each box equals 8oz.

Snack-Meal #4 _____

Snack-Meal #5 _____

Healthy Lean Meal   Protein   _____

2 Vegetables _____   Step Reading:_____

"Journaling is like whispering to one's self and listening at the same time."

~ Mina Murray

THE GOAL AND THE SOUL

Daily Goals

Write your goals in the space provided. These are your weight loss goals, your change-in-eating goals, your fitness and exercise goals and any other goals you want to achieve over time. Writing and re-writing goals daily is very powerful.

_____

_____

_____

_____

_____

_____

_____

Daily Soul
(Your Journal)

Write your feelings, thoughts and ideas below. These should include things you learned today, things you are excited about today, and things that you are grateful for today. Include any other details of the day you believe are important. This is your private workbook. Be honest with yourself. How do you really feel? Get it out of your head and on paper!

_____

_____

_____

_____

_____

What's Your Story
(Tasks and Victories)

"No, Doctor, I don't' want to grow young again. I just want to keep growing old."

~ Madame de Rothschild

DAY 15
Ketone Breath – Probably Not

Lesson:

Many people are concerned about developing bad breath while losing weight. On a highly ketogenic diet this may be the case. The ketones transfer to our breath and smell "funny." Remember, you are on a normal protein, reduced carbohydrate, controlled fat diet. You will experience only mild ketosis. Because of this, you will not have the common side effects of some of the popular severe carbohydrate restriction diets. If you are one of the few that do have bad breath problems on this program; and, if someone mentions it, just smile and thank them for noticing that you're burning fat. I doubt they mention it again.

If you do develop a change in your breath odor during your fat loss phase, there are several ways to deal with it. Drinking your water at regular intervals throughout the day will rinse your mouth and aid digestion. This has a positive effect on breath odor. Using a mild mouth-wash several times a day will also prove beneficial. Avoid frequent use of the highly-oxidizing mouthwashes as they may irritate the membranes of the mouth and tongue.

Brushing your teeth several times daily will keep your breath fresh and will also decrease a sudden hunger episode. There are several commercial mouth sprays available for use throughout the day. Be sure to check carbohydrate content of the spray, or rinse out your mouth after usage.

The most important thing to remember is that your body is burning fat and this process may temporarily change your breath odor. This will be minimized by making sure to eat six times daily. Now you can breathe easily.

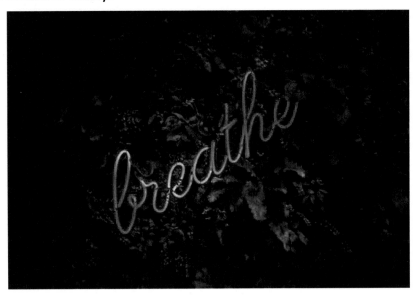

LEAN 51   DAILY TRACKER

Check off each item throughout the day to keep track of food, vitamins, water, and exercise.

Day # _____   Weight _____   Vitamin Pack _____

Your Daily Dietary Plan

Snack-Meal #1 _____   (Eat this first meal within 1 hour of arising)

Snack-Meal #2 _____

Snack-Meal #3 _____

Daily Fluid intake
each box equals 8oz.

Snack-Meal #4 _____

Snack-Meal #5 _____

Healthy Lean Meal   Protein   _____

2 Vegetables _____   Step Reading:_____

"Journaling is like whispering to one's self and lis-tening at the same time."

~ Mina Murray

THE GOAL AND THE SOUL

Daily Goals

Write your goals in the space provided. These are your weight loss goals, your change-in-eating goals, your fitness and exercise goals and any other goals you want to achieve over time. Writing and re-writing goals daily is very powerful.

_____

_____

_____

_____

_____

_____

Daily Soul
(Your Journal)

Write your feelings, thoughts and ideas below. These should include things you learned today, things you are excited about today, and things that you are grateful for today. Include any other details of the day you believe are important. This is your private workbook. Be honest with yourself. How do you really feel? Get it out of your head and on paper!

_____

_____

_____

_____

_____

_____

_____

What's Your Story
(Tasks and Victories)

_____

_____

_____

_____

_____

_____

_____

_____

_____

_____

"Strength is a matter of the made-up mind."

~ John Beecher

DAY 16
Watch the Right "Program"

Lesson:

A recent university study found that people who watch more than 2 hours of TV each night, have much greater rates if obesity. There are two overwhelming reasons for this. First, when we watch TV, we are sedentary. Our minds may be stimulated (occasionally), but our bodies are as relaxed as they have been all day. The other reason for television associated obesity is that we love to munch while we watch. We've all experienced eating while watching TV and at the end of the program, our snack bag or box was empty. "Where did all that food go?", runs through our mind. The truth – we ate it unconsciously.

To lose weight, decrease your TV time and take a walk, play with the kids, or participate in a hobby. Remember, when you do catch your favorite show, you are not allowed to visit the kitchen or pantry during the commercials. These same statistics apply to computer screen time. Be aware of how much time you sit in front of any screen. We are watching.

As reviewed earlier, the typical American diet is deficient in calories throughout the day and heavy in calories at night. When we have deprived ourselves of the necessary fuel in the morning and afternoon, our body encourages us to "catch up" in the evening. Many people will eat their evening meal (which is, unfortunately, the largest meal of the day) and be back in the kitchen or pantry within 1-2 hours for dessert or high-fat and carbohydrate snacks.

Be sure to use your protein snack meals in the evening to avoid these cravings. By consistently avoiding the late-night chips, popcorn, or ice cream, a new habit of healthy eating will energize and assist you in your fat loss process. This process is a reprogramming of your eating patterns. Your new eating program will be the best program you'll ever watch.

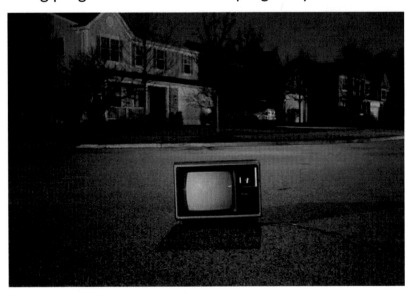

LEAN 51   DAILY TRACKER

Check off each item throughout the day to keep track of food, vitamins, water, and exercise.

Day # _____   Weight _____   Vitamin Pack _____

Your Daily Dietary Plan

Snack-Meal #1 _____   (Eat this first meal within 1 hour of arising)

Snack-Meal #2 _____

Daily Fluid intake
each box equals 8oz.

Snack-Meal #3 _____

Snack-Meal #4 _____

Snack-Meal #5 _____

Healthy Lean Meal   Protein   _____

2 Vegetables _____   Step Reading:_____

"Journaling is like whispering to one's self and listening at the same time."

~ Mina Murray

THE GOAL AND THE SOUL

Daily Goals

Write your goals in the space provided. These are your weight loss goals, your change-in-eating goals, your fitness and exercise goals and any other goals you want to achieve over time. Writing and re-writing goals daily is very powerful.

_____

_____

_____

_____

_____

_____

Daily Soul
(Your Journal)

Write your feelings, thoughts and ideas below. These should include things you learned today, things you are excited about today, and things that you are grateful for today. Include any other details of the day you believe are important. This is your private workbook. Be honest with yourself. How do you really feel? Get it out of your head and on paper!

_____

_____

_____

_____

_____

_____

_____

What's Your Story
(Tasks and Victories)

_____

_____

_____

_____

_____

_____

_____

_____

_____

_____

"Knowing is not enough, we must apply. Willing is not enough, we must do."

~ Johann von Goethe

DAY 17
Keep on Logging

Lesson:

Using the check-off sheet every day helps to develop a strong habit. Don't ignore this simple tool. It keeps you focused on your daily plan. It adds to your sense of discipline and accomplishment. When you do eat something not on the program and you list it, you have just given yourself a dietary lesson. When we write down everything we eat, we become aware of the bad habits. It becomes much easier to replace a bad habit with a good one when we are aware of it. Writing down your daily "steps total" from the step tracker will help you reach your activity goal.

Recording your daily weight makes this program a priority in your life. Staying in touch with your team members involves you in something more important than each of us individually. You'll be more likely to not miss the vitamins and supplements when you check them off. Finally, be sure to write down your daily thoughts. A mentor of mine once said, "if your life is worth living, it's worth writing about."

Each day of this manual is designed to be repetitious. The daily repetition develops a pattern that will be easy to follow the rest of your life. If you play a musical instrument well, you learned it through daily repetition of the basics. You played scales and notes over and over until you no longer needed to think about them. Riding a bicycle, golfing, skiing, and all other complex activities can be learned through repetitive practice of certain individual tasks or skills.

Learning the LEAN 51 lifestyle is nothing more than mastering certain dietary and exercise tasks and skills. Be excited about the simplicity of these tasks and skills and repeat them over and over until you don't have to think about them anymore. Being LEAN will be a part of who you are.

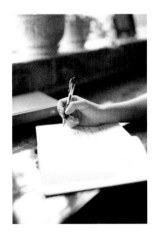

LEAN 51   DAILY TRACKER

Check off each item throughout the day to keep track of food, vitamins, water, and exercise.

Day # _____   Weight _____   Vitamin Pack _____

Your Daily Dietary Plan

Snack-Meal #1 _____   (Eat this first meal within 1 hour of arising)

Snack-Meal #2 _____

Snack-Meal #3 _____

Daily Fluid intake
each box equals 8oz.

Snack-Meal #4 _____

Snack-Meal #5 _____

Healthy Lean Meal   Protein   _____

2 Vegetables _____   Step Reading:_____

"Journaling is like whispering to one's self and listening at the same time."

~ Mina Murray

THE GOAL AND THE SOUL

Daily Goals

Write your goals in the space provided. These are your weight loss goals, your change-in-eating goals, your fitness and exercise goals and any other goals you want to achieve over time. Writing and re-writing goals daily is very powerful.

_____

_____

_____

_____

_____

_____

Daily Soul
(Your Journal)

Write your feelings, thoughts and ideas below. These should include things you learned today, things you are excited about today, and things that you are grateful for today. Include any other details of the day you believe are important. This is your private workbook. Be honest with yourself. How do you really feel? Get it out of your head and on paper!

_____

_____

_____

_____

_____

_____

_____

What's Your Story
(Tasks and Victories)

_____

_____

_____

_____

_____

_____

_____

_____

_____

_____

"Nothing can be done except little by little."

~ Charles Bandelaire

DAY 18
Be Nice to Yourself

Lesson:

We eat for many reasons and it's usually not for nutritional support. We eat when we are bored. We eat when we are lonely. We eat to celebrate and to socialize. We eat when we feel down and we eat when we're stressed. I bet you can think of other reasons why you eat. Uncovering the reasons you eat will assist you on your weight loss journey. When we eat as a form of relief or reward, we only feel better until we swallow. Keep track of when you think of food. Work toward finding your eating triggers. Breaking these patterns may require additional help. If you suffer from "Food Therapy" let us know.

We can recommend several good books or even a counselor. We now have a psychologic evaluation called the "Inner Diet" developed by Dr. John Sklane. Be sure to take the evaluation and then go through the cognitive and behavior modification program supplied as part of LEAN 51. Eating is primarily the way our body gets its fuel. Yes, it should be tasty and a pleasant experience, but it is not the answer to life's concerns. If you learn to deal with this, you will live a leaner, longer, and healthier life!

As you eliminate food as a drug in your life, you will need to replace it with a more healthful substitute. Addiction counselors and therapists help alcohol and drug addicts to find healthier methods to alleviate stressful situations. The same is true for food overuse. Instead of eating to calm or soothe yourself, find another activity which will provide similar results. Meditation, exercise, reading, or contacting an accountability partner can be great substitutes. Many of our LEAN 51 partners pair up and hold each other accountable.

When life throws us a curve ball and we become stressed, call your partner for help. I recommend establishing a pact with a fellow "fat loser" and make sure the accountability is based on trust, honesty, and true concern for each other. Be encouraging and supportive of each other. By being helpful and nice to someone else, you will learn to be helpful and nice to yourself. If you don't have someone to work with, our health coaches are here for you. They're nice also!

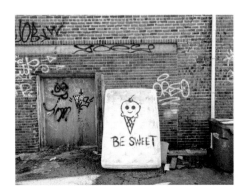

LEAN 51   DAILY TRACKER

Check off each item throughout the day to keep track of food, vitamins, water, and exercise.

Day # _____   Weight _____   Vitamin Pack _____

Your Daily Dietary Plan

Snack-Meal #1 _____   (Eat this first meal within 1 hour of arising)

Snack-Meal #2 _____

Snack-Meal #3 _____   **Daily Fluid intake**

Snack-Meal #4 _____   each box equals 8oz.

Snack-Meal #5 _____

Healthy Lean Meal   Protein   _____

                    2 Vegetables _____   Step Reading:_____

"Journaling is like whispering to one's self and listening at the same time."

~ Mina Murray

THE GOAL AND THE SOUL

Daily Goals

Write your goals in the space provided. These are your weight loss goals, your change-in-eating goals, your fitness and exercise goals and any other goals you want to achieve over time. Writing and re-writing goals daily is very powerful.

_____

_____

_____

_____

_____

_____

Daily Soul
(Your Journal)

Write your feelings, thoughts and ideas below. These should include things you learned today, things you are excited about today, and things that you are grateful for today. Include any other details of the day you believe are important. This is your private workbook. Be honest with yourself. How do you really feel? Get it out of your head and on paper!

_____

_____

_____

_____

_____

_____

_____

What's Your Story
(Tasks and Victories)

_____

_____

_____

_____

_____

_____

_____

_____

_____

_____

"If you want something, do it!"

~ Plautus

DAY 19
Are Carbs Really the Enemy?

Lesson:

Carbohydrates, proteins, and fats are necessary for life. Carbohydrates come in two forms; refined and unrefined. Refined carbohydrates are the processed sugars and flours. These are less healthy for us. Unrefined carbohydrates are the ones found in whole grains, fruits, beans, and most vegetables. All carbohydrates are eventually broken down in your body to glucose (your blood sugar). The reason carbohydrates present a problem is that eating more than we can use causes the remaining excess glucose to be converted to fat.

Eating lots of candy, cookies, soft drinks, chips and sweets produces a cycle of excess glucose and fat creation. Controlling the amount of carbohydrates we eat to between 100 – 150 grams. or less, daily during the dietary plan prevents formation of new fat and stimulates breakdown of our fat storage. Reducing refined carbohydrates and using unrefined carbo-hydrates in limited quantities will ensure long-term weight maintenance. You'll soon be a "Health Addict," not a "Carb Addict."

Many people wonder if they will ever be able to eat a dessert or carbohydrate-laden food again. The answer is yes. Learning how to incorporate carbohydrates of this type into your diet will not be difficult. As you lose fat, become stronger and more fit, your body will process and burn carbohydrates more effectively. You will be able to eat small amounts of these foods in your lifetime maintenance plan. You will learn to eat at the right times in the right quanti-ties. You will enjoy them as part of your diet, but not let them interfere with your health ever again. You will be disciplined by your control over fat-producing foods. You will be master of your body. You will focus on foods that sustain your good health. You will eat to live, not live to eat.

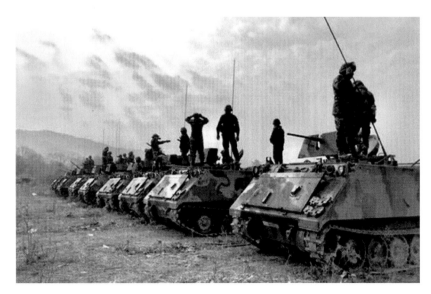

LEAN 51   DAILY TRACKER

Check off each item throughout the day to keep track of food, vitamins, water, and exercise.

Day # _____   Weight _____   Vitamin Pack _____

Your Daily Dietary Plan

Snack-Meal #1 _____   (Eat this first meal within 1 hour of arising)

Snack-Meal #2 _____

Snack-Meal #3 _____   **Daily Fluid intake**

each box equals 8oz.

Snack-Meal #4 _____

Snack-Meal #5 _____

Healthy Lean Meal   Protein   _____

2 Vegetables _____   Step Reading:_____

"Journaling is like whispering to one's self and listening at the same time."

~ Mina Murray

THE GOAL AND THE SOUL

Daily Goals

Write your goals in the space provided. These are your weight loss goals, your change-in-eating goals, your fitness and exercise goals and any other goals you want to achieve over time. Writing and re-writing goals daily is very powerful.

_____

_____

_____

_____

_____

_____

_____

Daily Soul
(Your Journal)

Write your feelings, thoughts and ideas below. These should include things you learned today, things you are excited about today, and things that you are grateful for today. Include any other details of the day you believe are important. This is your private workbook. Be honest with yourself. How do you really feel? Get it out of your head and on paper!

_____

_____

_____

_____

_____

_____

_____

<u>What's Your Story</u>
(Tasks and Victories)

_____

_____

_____

_____

_____

_____

_____

_____

_____

_____

_____

"Happiness lies, first of all, in health."

~ George William Curtis

DAY 20
Take Your Supplements

Lesson:

Although vitamins, minerals, and essential fatty acids are not truly medicines, they are extremely beneficial to achieve optimum health. Our patients tell us that they feel better and have more energy when they include the daily multi-vitamin and Omega 3 fatty acids in their program.

Patients often ask if vitamins are necessary. My answer is if you eat a well-balanced healthful diet, get adequate exercise, have no stress, get sufficient sleep, avoid all toxins such as smoking and alcohol and have excess energy every day, you don't need them. While losing weight the body is activating several processes. The daily supplements will protect your body from developing any deficiencies as you physically change to a lean and fit you. So, take your supplements like a good boy or girl.

Vitamins are substances that our body requires to perform the chemical reactions necessary for health. Some vitamins assist in the formation of new cells and tissues. Some work to help produce energy using amino acids, which are the building blocks of proteins. Certain vitamins are needed for good vision and healthy skin. Other vitamins continue to be part of molecules necessary for growth and tissue regeneration.

We get the majority of vitamins from our food intake. The LEAN 51 program provides a nutritious diet that provides for an adequate supply of vitamins. The added vitamin supplement is an insurance policy while your body is converting to fat reduction and muscle sparing activities. Don't miss your daily vitamin pack. You'll be glad you did.

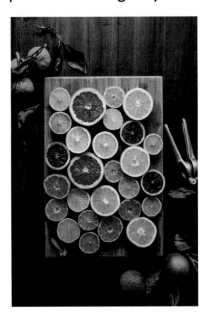

LEAN 51   DAILY TRACKER

Check off each item throughout the day to keep track of food, vitamins, water, and exercise.

Day # _____   Weight _____   Vitamin Pack _____

Your Daily Dietary Plan

Snack-Meal #1 _____   (Eat this first meal within 1 hour of arising)

Snack-Meal #2 _____

Daily Fluid intake
each box equals 8oz.

Snack-Meal #3 _____

Snack-Meal #4 _____

Snack-Meal #5 _____

Healthy Lean Meal   Protein   _____

2 Vegetables _____   Step Reading:_____

"Journaling is like whispering to one's self and listening at the same time."

~ Mina Murray

THE GOAL AND THE SOUL

Daily Goals

Write your goals in the space provided. These are your weight loss goals, your change-in-eating goals, your fitness and exercise goals and any other goals you want to achieve over time. Writing and re-writing goals daily is very powerful.

_____

_____

_____

_____

_____

_____

_____

Daily Soul
(Your Journal)

Write your feelings, thoughts and ideas below. These should include things you learned today, things you are excited about today, and things that you are grateful for today. Include any other details of the day you believe are important. This is your private workbook. Be honest with yourself. How do you really feel? Get it out of your head and on paper!

_____

_____

_____

_____

_____

_____

_____

What's Your Story
(Tasks and Victories)

_____

_____

_____

_____

_____

_____

_____

_____

_____

_____

"Be like a postage stamp – stick to one think until you get there."

~ Josh Billings

DAY 21
The Dreaded Plateau

Lesson:

It would be wonderful if every day when we stepped on the scale another pound dropped off. That's just not reality. As we work to change our body's way of functioning, we all will encounter resistance. When our body resists weight loss, we call this a plateau. In fact, it is quite normal to lose pounds in a stair step fashion. This allows time for our tissue and chemical processes to adjust to our new way of life. Yes, the plateau is frustrating, but I like to think it's our body's way of saying "I'm not sure you are committed to losing this weight." When you prove your commitment by sticking with the program, you are always rewarded with more weight loss.

Sometimes plateaus are the result of water retention. Some theories suggest that water temporarily replaces rapidly lost fat and this is eliminated as the fat cell restructures its size. Since water weighs more than fat, the scale doesn't budge. Whether true or not, it's a reasonable way to explain your plateaus and help get through them. Remember, when climbing a mountain, reaching a plateau is not such a bad place for a while.

The greatest risk to someone who is attempting to become healthy is frustration. Many dietary programs have been abandoned from one single frustrating day. At times, the frustrations may be set off by someone who criticizes us. It amazes me that the same people who say we are fat or overweight behind our backs are the first ones to tell us our diet is wrong or we're losing too fast or one sweet snack or dessert won't hurt us.

When you change your life for the better, others may be upset because you have caused them to look at their own lives. If they don't like what they see, you may be the one they blame. Stand strong and firm that you are on the right path and that your life is at stake. Be the example for others and let them make their own decisions about their lifestyle. You will soon be standing tall on the mountain of success. You will have overcome every plateau and every frustration.

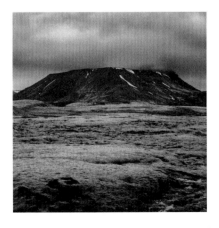

LEAN 51   DAILY TRACKER

Check off each item throughout the day to keep track of food, vitamins, water, and exercise.

Day # _____   Weight _____   Vitamin Pack _____

Your Daily Dietary Plan

Snack-Meal #1 _____   (Eat this first meal within 1 hour of arising)

Snack-Meal #2 _____

Snack-Meal #3 _____   **Daily Fluid intake**

Snack-Meal #4 _____   each box equals 8oz.

Snack-Meal #5 _____

Healthy Lean Meal   Protein   _____

2 Vegetables _____   Step Reading:_____

"Journaling is like whispering to one's self and listening at the same time."

~ Mina Murray

THE GOAL AND THE SOUL

Daily Goals

Write your goals in the space provided. These are your weight loss goals, your change-in-eating goals, your fitness and exercise goals and any other goals you want to achieve over time. Writing and re-writing goals daily is very powerful.

_____

_____

_____

_____

_____

_____

_____

Daily Soul
(Your Journal)

Write your feelings, thoughts and ideas below. These should include things you learned today, things you are excited about today, and things that you are grateful for today. Include any other details of the day you believe are important. This is your private workbook. Be honest with yourself. How do you really feel? Get it out of your head and on paper!

_____

_____

_____

_____

_____

_____

_____

What's Your Story
(Tasks and Victories)

_____

_____

_____

_____

_____

_____

_____

_____

_____

_____

"It does not matter how slowly you go, so long as you do not stop."

DAY 22
Motion Improves Emotion

Lesson:

By this time, you have been on the program for 3 weeks. You have dropped a moderate amount of weight. The energy you feel is a great benefit. The numbers of steps are growing more easily. Many people feel like increasing their activity level at this point. There are many great ways to expand the physical activity and exercise that will be important for long-term weight control and improved health. Here are several ideas to help you become less sedentary and more active.

- Take the stairs instead of the elevator
- Park further away from stores and buildings
- Join a health club or gym – and use it
- Take an exercise class; beginner classes are usually available to start out with
- Hire a personal trainer
- Exercise with a friend or family member
- Set realistic goals to prevent soreness and injury
- Work in the yard
- Walk the golf course instead of using a cart
- Take trips to the mall and walk from end to end
- Be sure to wear proper shoes
- Schedule exercise into your daily planner

Remember, a good exercise habit will help you stay leaner the rest of your life. An extra benefit of increased physical activity is that "Motion improves Emotion," so exercise and be happy!

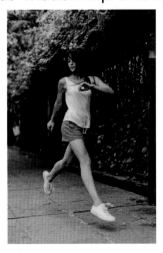

LEAN 51   DAILY TRACKER

Check off each item throughout the day to keep track of food, vitamins, water, and exercise.

Day # _____   Weight _____   Vitamin Pack _____

Your Daily Dietary Plan

Snack-Meal #1 _____   (Eat this first meal within 1 hour of arising)

Snack-Meal #2 _____

Snack-Meal #3 _____   **Daily Fluid intake**

each box equals 8oz.

Snack-Meal #4 _____

Snack-Meal #5 _____

Healthy Lean Meal   Protein   _____

2 Vegetables _____   Step Reading:_____

"Journaling is like whispering to one's self and listening at the same time."

~ Mina Murray

THE GOAL AND THE SOUL

Daily Goals

Write your goals in the space provided. These are your weight loss goals, your change-in-eating goals, your fitness and exercise goals and any other goals you want to achieve over time. Writing and re-writing goals daily is very powerful.

_____

_____

_____

_____

_____

_____

_____

Daily Soul
(Your Journal)

Write your feelings, thoughts and ideas below. These should include things you learned today, things you are excited about today, and things that you are grateful for today. Include any other details of the day you believe are important. This is your private workbook. Be honest with yourself. How do you really feel? Get it out of your head and on paper!

_____

_____

_____

_____

_____

What's Your Story
(Tasks and Victories)

"We can do anything we want to do if we stick to it long enough."

~ Helen Keller

DAY 23
Break the Habit

Lesson:

The LEAN 51 program is about creating new habits. There are many factors that have caused you to be overweight. Some hereditary or genetic patterns for obesity are felt to be causes. Our environment, or how our parents ate and taught us to eat, has played a major role. Our behavior patterns and how we use food for non-nutritional purposes promotes obesity. Commercial advertising and suggestive marketing pulls us toward high fat, high carbohydrate foods.

Over the years, these complex factors have all contributed to your weight gain. To continue to lose weight and maintain a lean body, new habits must be created. As many have said, "If you keep doing what you're doing, you will keep getting what you're getting." If you want to change your life, you have to change your thinking. The LEAN 51 Plan is designed to change how you think about food, eating, nutrition, exercise, and overall health. By doing the daily tasks, following the menus and logging your progress, you are retraining your brain to follow a new pattern. You are learning the "LEAN 51 Pattern."

By now, you could probably teach the LEAN 51 Program to someone else. This is a good sign you are committed to turning the plan from a step-by-step program to a lifelong pattern. As you lose weight, you may be asked how you are doing it. This is a good opportunity to see how well you understand and know the program. Don't be a salesperson, but try to explain the program to this person in your own words. You will be amazed at what you've learned so far.

Your personal experience on the program is an educational program in itself. It's been known for centuries that we learn best by explaining and teaching others. Use these opportunities to more deeply learn the LEAN 51 Program. If your questioner is interested in becoming healthier, you can let our coaches answer their additional questions.

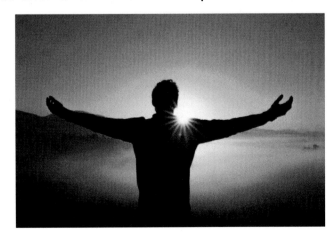

LEAN 51   DAILY TRACKER

Check off each item throughout the day to keep track of food, vitamins, water, and exercise.

Day # _____   Weight _____   Vitamin Pack _____

Your Daily Dietary Plan

Snack-Meal #1 _____   (Eat this first meal within 1 hour of arising)

Snack-Meal #2 _____

Daily Fluid intake

Snack-Meal #3 _____   each box equals 8oz.

Snack-Meal #4 _____

Snack-Meal #5 _____

Healthy Lean Meal   Protein   _____

                      2 Vegetables _____   Step Reading:_____

"Journaling is like whispering to one's self and listening at the same time."

~ Mina Murray

THE GOAL AND THE SOUL

Daily Goals

Write your goals in the space provided. These are your weight loss goals, your change-in-eating goals, your fitness and exercise goals and any other goals you want to achieve over time. Writing and re-writing goals daily is very powerful.

_____

_____

_____

_____

_____

_____

_____

Daily Soul
(Your Journal)

Write your feelings, thoughts and ideas below. These should include things you learned today, things you are excited about today, and things that you are grateful for today. Include any other details of the day you believe are important. This is your private workbook. Be honest with yourself. How do you really feel? Get it out of your head and on paper!

_____

_____

_____

_____

_____

What's Your Story
(Tasks and Victories)

Too many people miss the silver lining because they're expecting gold."

~ Maurice Setter

DAY 24
Food is Fuel

Lesson:

Food is abundant and easy to get our hands on. Because of this, we must begin to think of food as fuel for our body. Our body requires a steady supply of fuel from a balanced diet. I like to think of my car and its need for fuel to help explain what our bodies need. We wouldn't get in our car to go somewhere and give the engine one big gulp of gas and expect to get very far. We also wouldn't deprive the engine of gas and be on our way. When we arise in the morning our body needs fuel. Breakfast is essential to getting our "engine" running right.

The LEAN 51 program provides a steady fuel source for our bodies by giving us food in appropriate quantities 6 times a day. Eating the right things at the right time allows for the smooth function of our systems, just like a steady step on the gas pedal allows our car to operate in a smooth efficient fashion.

Avoid the unconscious eating, the nighttime munchies, the starvation periods and binges, by sticking closely to the meal plan and menu. Avoid eating while watching TV. Stop skipping meals. Think of your body as a lean machine and give it the recommended fuel supply for its most efficient operation.

The human body is designed to store fuel as fat when there is an abundance of calories. When there is a deficiency of food our body is very efficient at slowing down the metabolism and using its reserve calorie stores wisely.

The LEAN 51 Program tells the body that there is enough fuel to keep the metabolism up, but not enough to store fat. Instead, the body senses a lack of fast glucose-producing foods and dips directly into its fat reserve to provide energy. This is how food is utilized while on this program. Our muscles and proteins are spared because we are supplying our body with adequate protein meals. Losing the fat and feeling healthy are accomplished simultaneously.

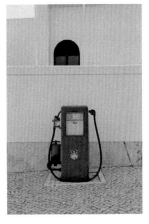

LEAN 51   DAILY TRACKER

Check off each item throughout the day to keep track of food, vitamins, water, and exercise.

Day # _____ Weight _____ Vitamin Pack _____

Your Daily Dietary Plan

Snack-Meal #1 _____   (Eat this first meal within 1 hour of arising)

Snack-Meal #2 _____

Snack-Meal #3 _____   **Daily Fluid intake**
each box equals 8oz.

Snack-Meal #4 _____

Snack-Meal #5 _____

Healthy Lean Meal   Protein   _____

2 Vegetables _____   Step Reading:_____

"Journaling is like whispering to one's self and listening at the same time."

~ Mina Murray

THE GOAL AND THE SOUL

Daily Goals

Write your goals in the space provided. These are your weight loss goals, your change-in-eating goals, your fitness and exercise goals and any other goals you want to achieve over time. Writing and re-writing goals daily is very powerful.

_____

_____

_____

_____

_____

_____

_____

Daily Soul
(Your Journal)

Write your feelings, thoughts and ideas below. These should include things you learned today, things you are excited about today, and things that you are grateful for today. Include any other details of the day you believe are important. This is your private workbook. Be honest with yourself. How do you really feel? Get it out of your head and on paper!

_____

_____

_____

_____

_____

_____

_____

<u>What's Your Story</u>
(Tasks and Victories)

_____

_____

_____

_____

_____

_____

_____

_____

_____

_____

"All I can say about life is, Oh God, enjoy it!"

~ Bob Newhart

DAY 25

Reward Yourself: You are closing in on a month of living healthy on the LEAN 51 Program.

Lesson:

In five more days you will reach a major milestone. For some, you will be ready for the Maintenance program. For others, you will want to continue losing weight. When you finish the first month, you need to reward yourself. By now, I hope your thinking has changed and you're not looking to reward yourself with a high-carbohydrate or high-fat trophy. That would be counterproductive. The best rewards are simple and meaningful. This would be a great time to congratulate yourself by taking your spouse, a friend, or family member to a movie. Take a snack meal with you.

A trip to the park or the beach, depending on where you live, would be a great way to spend a day and get some extra physical activity. Think of something fun and easy you like to do and plan it as a celebration of your month-long commitment. It's also a good time to write down your goals for the next 30 days and put another reward on the page so you have a second commendation awaiting you. If you're like most people, you feel like you have come very far, yet also realize that you're just beginning. Your biggest reward will be improved health, extra energy, and the satisfaction you have deep down inside knowing you are in control of your life.

It is the desire of everyone to feel healthy, happy and to accomplish something important. Becoming fit and lean will create a positive spirit within you. Many of our team members say that losing the fat and closing in on their optimum weight loss has given them a new perspective on life. They feel happier. They feel confident. They feel a strong sense of personal achievement. These positive feelings carry over into other areas of their lives.

They comment about improved work habits, better relationships and the ability to control other life problems. It is very common for the power we get from focus and commitment in one area of life to create a positive spillover into our entire life. Keep focused and give yourself a pat on the back. You've done well.

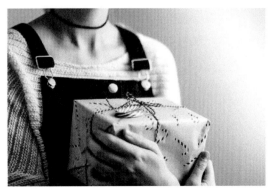

LEAN 51   DAILY TRACKER

Check off each item throughout the day to keep track of food, vitamins, water, and exercise.

Day # _____   Weight _____   Vitamin Pack _____

Your Daily Dietary Plan

Snack-Meal #1 _____   (Eat this first meal within 1 hour of arising)

Snack-Meal #2 _____

Snack-Meal #3 _____   ## Daily Fluid intake

Snack-Meal #4 _____   each box equals 8oz.

Snack-Meal #5 _____

Healthy Lean Meal   Protein   _____

                              2 Vegetables _____   Step Reading:_____

"Journaling is like whispering to one's self and listening at the same time."

~ Mina Murray

THE GOAL AND THE SOUL

Daily Goals

Write your goals in the space provided. These are your weight loss goals, your change-in-eating goals, your fitness and exercise goals and any other goals you want to achieve over time. Writing and re-writing goals daily is very powerful.

_____

_____

_____

_____

_____

_____

_____

Daily Soul
(Your Journal)

Write your feelings, thoughts and ideas below. These should include things you learned today, things you are excited about today, and things that you are grateful for today. Include any other details of the day you believe are important. This is your private workbook. Be honest with yourself. How do you really feel? Get it out of your head and on paper!

_____

_____

_____

_____

_____

_____

_____

<u>What's Your Story</u>
(Tasks and Victories)

_____

_____

_____

_____

_____

_____

_____

_____

_____

_____

"Life is 10 percent what you make it and 90 percent how you take it."

~ Irving Berlin

DAY 26
Metabolism

Lesson:

As you lose weight, and especially fat, your body has a built-in safety mechanism to gradually slow down its metabolism. This is a protection against starvation. Without food, we slow our functions down to conserve our tissues. With the LEAN 51 Program, this tendency is blunted, but your metabolic rate does slow mildly. In calorie deprivation diets, most people would feel extremely tired and cold most of the time after 4 weeks. If you've experienced this, then you may not be eating enough. Sometimes our history of dieting the wrong way sneaks back up on us and we subconsciously eat too little.

The LEAN 51 Program requires that you eat 6 times a day. The increase in steps you have tracked on your step tracker has helped to keep your metabolic rate up. Continue to increase your steps slowly and surely. If you are someone who needs to lose more than 40 pounds, it is important to keep your metabolic rate up by eating every 3 hours and getting in your daily steps. An analogy would be that of a water heater.

Every water heater has a layer of insulation in it. If we take off the insulation jacket, it takes more heat and therefore, more fuel to keep the water hot. In our body, as we lose weight, we remove our insulation jacket. It then takes more energy or fuel to keep our body warm and functioning well. Compared to the day you started on LEAN 51, your blood sugar is now more stable, your cholesterol is better, your blood pressure is lower and you are more fit. You are stronger and just feel better. Keep up the great work!

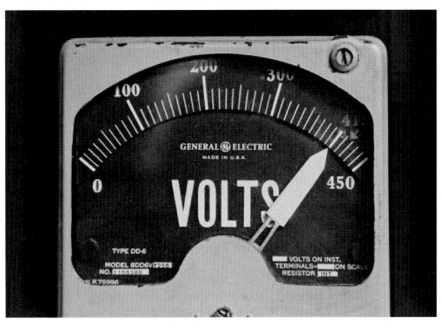

LEAN 51   DAILY TRACKER

Check off each item throughout the day to keep track of food, vitamins, water, and exercise.

Day # _____   Weight _____   Vitamin Pack _____

Your Daily Dietary Plan

Snack-Meal #1 _____   (Eat this first meal within 1 hour of arising)

Snack-Meal #2 _____

Snack-Meal #3 _____   **Daily Fluid intake**

Snack-Meal #4 _____   each box equals 8oz.

Snack-Meal #5 _____

Healthy Lean Meal   Protein   _____

2 Vegetables _____   Step Reading:_____

"Journaling is like whispering to one's self and lis-tening at the same time."

~ Mina Murray

THE GOAL AND THE SOUL

Daily Goals

Write your goals in the space provided. These are your weight loss goals, your change-in-eating goals, your fitness and exercise goals and any other goals you want to achieve over time. Writing and re-writing goals daily is very powerful.

_____

_____

_____

_____

_____

_____

_____

Daily Soul
(Your Journal)

Write your feelings, thoughts and ideas below. These should include things you learned today, things you are excited about today, and things that you are grateful for today. Include any other details of the day you believe are important. This is your private workbook. Be honest with yourself. How do you really feel? Get it out of your head and on paper!

_____

_____

_____

_____

_____

_____

_____

What's Your Story
(Tasks and Victories)

_____

_____

_____

_____

_____

_____

_____

_____

_____

_____

"The pursuit of happiness...is the greatest feat man has to accomplish."

~ Robert Henri

DAY 27
Stay in Touch

Lesson:

I get e-mail from team members every day. It's exciting to hear from them and to get progress reports on their weight loss. I have received new ideas from team members that have enhanced our program. Sometimes, I get important questions and other times I get a weight loss total-to-date. Often I get a communication where someone just needs a bit of encouragement. We all need encouragement on a regular basis. If you are a little on the shy side and haven't sent me an e-mail, make it a priority to get in touch. Not only will you get a lift, but so will I.

It's a great feeling for me to learn that you are working toward your health goals and making progress. An important feature of the LEAN 51 Program that most other programs don't have is that you are not required to attend meetings or weigh-ins. You can be as independent as you like. Studies do confirm that people who have a support system in place, and use it, lose more weight, and maintain weight loss better. Let us be your support system. So send us an e-mail, you just might make our day!

Our email is fatdocthindoc@gmail.com . When I played sports, I always became better when a coach took time to assist and encourage me. Today there are coaching and mentoring programs available through many organizations. On our LEAN plans, we feel that a coach plays a valuable role in our treatment. It encourages you to work with your weight loss coach on a regular basis.

The coach is someone who understands the LEAN 51 Program and lives at their desired weight. They are personally living a healthy life and can assist you with goal setting, accountability, and encouragement. So while you're on the team, take advantage of the coach. I know that you and your coach will have a winning season.

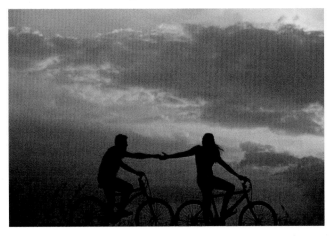

LEAN 51   DAILY TRACKER

Check off each item throughout the day to keep track of food, vitamins, water, and exercise.

Day # _____   Weight _____   Vitamin Pack _____

Your Daily Dietary Plan

Snack-Meal #1 _____   (Eat this first meal within 1 hour of arising)

Snack-Meal #2 _____

Snack-Meal #3 _____   ## Daily Fluid intake
                                   each box equals 8oz.
Snack-Meal #4 _____

Snack-Meal #5 _____

Healthy Lean Meal   Protein   _____

                      2 Vegetables _____   Step Reading:_____

"Journaling is like whispering to one's self and listening at the same time."

~ Mina Murray

THE GOAL AND THE SOUL

Daily Goals

Write your goals in the space provided. These are your weight loss goals, your change-in-eating goals, your fitness and exercise goals and any other goals you want to achieve over time. Writing and re-writing goals daily is very powerful.

_____

_____

_____

_____

_____

_____

Daily Soul
(Your Journal)

Write your feelings, thoughts and ideas below. These should include things you learned today, things you are excited about today, and things that you are grateful for today. Include any other details of the day you believe are important. This is your private workbook. Be honest with yourself. How do you really feel? Get it out of your head and on paper!

_____

_____

_____

_____

_____

_____

_____

What's Your Story
(Tasks and Victories)

_____

_____

_____

_____

_____

_____

_____

_____

_____

_____

"Most folks are about as happy as they make up their minds to be."

~ Abraham Lincoln

DAY 28
Eating Out - Safely

Lesson:

Americans are eating more and more meals in restaurants. In almost every moderate or larger-sized city, main streets are lined with restaurants. When I started the program for myself, I knew that eating meals in restaurants could be my downfall. What I discovered was the LEAN 51 plan was perfect for almost every restaurant. What restaurant can't supply you with a lean protein (chicken, fish, turkey or beef), a salad, and vegetables? I found nearly all of them can.

In my second month on the program, I spent 7 days in a hotel in downtown Boston at a medical conference. I ate supper at a restaurant each day. With a minimal amount of searching, I was able to find reasonably priced meals that fit my program perfectly and lost 3 pounds that week.

Many restaurant menus have low-fat salads with lean meats on them. These can serve as a whole meal. Just be careful to watch the dressings. Limit dressings by using only 1 tablespoon full. If you like lots of dressing, try adding a packet of sugar substitute to your salad and mix it up. It's usually the sweetness we are looking for. You must prepare your mind when you enter the restaurant to avoid the bowl of rolls, the specials of the day and the desserts. You can do it – Plan it and give it a try.

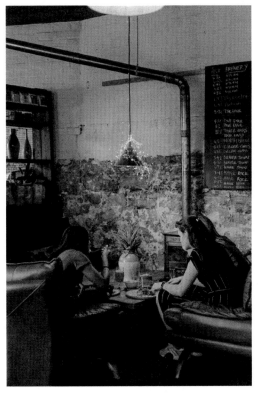

LEAN 51   DAILY TRACKER

Check off each item throughout the day to keep track of food, vitamins, water, and exercise.

Day # _____   Weight _____   Vitamin Pack _____

Your Daily Dietary Plan

Snack-Meal #1 _____   (Eat this first meal within 1 hour of arising)

Snack-Meal #2 _____

Snack-Meal #3 _____   **Daily Fluid intake**

Snack-Meal #4 _____   each box equals 8oz.

Snack-Meal #5 _____

Healthy Lean Meal   Protein   _____

                      2 Vegetables _____   Step Reading:_____

"Journaling is like whispering to one's self and listening at the same time."

~ Mina Murray

THE GOAL AND THE SOUL

Daily Goals

Write your goals in the space provided. These are your weight loss goals, your change-in-eating goals, your fitness and exercise goals and any other goals you want to achieve over time. Writing and re-writing goals daily is very powerful.

_____

_____

_____

_____

_____

_____

_____

Daily Soul
(Your Journal)

Write your feelings, thoughts and ideas below. These should include things you learned today, things you are excited about today, and things that you are grateful for today. Include any other details of the day you believe are important. This is your private workbook. Be honest with yourself. How do you really feel? Get it out of your head and on paper!

_____

_____

_____

_____

_____

What's Your Story
(Tasks and Victories)

"We must accept finite disappointment, but we must never lose infinite hope."

~ Martin Luther King, Jr.

DAY 29
Positive Thoughts – Positive Questions

Lesson:

Throughout the entire day, you are having a conversation with yourself. You silently ask yourself questions and you always receive a silent answer. Your brain was programmed to carry on this discussion as a way to learn, expand thoughts, find solutions, develop patterns and experience our surroundings. As we go through our daily routine, our conscious mind evaluates, thinks and responds.

Most of our experiences are funneled deeper into the subconscious mind for later remembrance, comparison, short-cuts or answers to questions and problems. Your subconscious mind remembers how you talk to yourself. As you go through your day, be nice to yourself. Don't ever say to yourself "I'm stupid", "I'm fat", or "I'm not deserving." Make a list of things you want to say to yourself like "I'm unique", "I'm responsible", or "I'm important to others." You will think of many positive, uplifting thoughts to tell yourself. Try it.

As for questions, avoid the unanswerable "Why?" question. Eliminate asking "Why me?", "Why did I do that?", or "Why can't I?" Instead, begin to ask "How?" questions to yourself. Such as "How can I eat out and stay on the program?", "How can I incorporate exercise into my busy schedule?", or "How do I enjoy every day on the LEAN 51 Program?" Your subconscious will give you great answers. So think better thoughts and ask better questions every day. Start today!

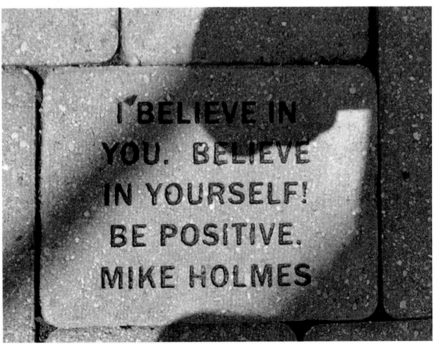

LEAN 51   DAILY TRACKER

Check off each item throughout the day to keep track of food, vitamins, water, and exercise.

Day # _____   Weight _____   Vitamin Pack _____

Your Daily Dietary Plan

Snack-Meal #1 _____   (Eat this first meal within 1 hour of arising)

Snack-Meal #2 _____

Snack-Meal #3 _____   **Daily Fluid intake**
                                 each box equals 8oz.

Snack-Meal #4 _____

Snack-Meal #5 _____

Healthy Lean Meal   Protein   _____

                 2 Vegetables _____   Step Reading:_____

"Journaling is like whispering to one's self and listening at the same time."

~ Mina Murray

THE GOAL AND THE SOUL

Daily Goals

Write your goals in the space provided. These are your weight loss goals, your change-in-eating goals, your fitness and exercise goals and any other goals you want to achieve over time. Writing and re-writing goals daily is very powerful.

_____

_____

_____

_____

_____

_____

_____

Daily Soul
(Your Journal)

Write your feelings, thoughts and ideas below. These should include things you learned today, things you are excited about today, and things that you are grateful for today. Include any other details of the day you believe are important. This is your private workbook. Be honest with yourself. How do you really feel? Get it out of your head and on paper!

_____

_____

_____

_____

_____

_____

_____

What's Your Story
(Tasks and Victories)

_____

_____

_____

_____

_____

_____

_____

_____

_____

"While you fear missing a meal, you aren't fully aware of meals you do eat."

~ Dan Millman

DAY 30
What a Difference 4 Weeks Can Make

Lesson:

When people decide to join our team and begin the LEAN 51 Program, they usually express many feelings. One feeling is that of excitement. The other feeling is doubt. Each of us has a small voice in our head that tells us we probably can't do this. Today, you can say "I did it." Though you aren't finished with the program, you have completed the first month of "fat loss." I believe that anyone who can commit and stay with this program for 4 weeks has learned the habits of LEAN 51.

New habits can be formed over a 21-25 day period, according to most psychologists. You have learned a great deal about yourself and you now know that you can live a healthier, longer, and leaner life. Many family members, friends, and acquaintances may now see a big difference in your appearance, your attitude and your lifestyle.

You are doing the opposite of the majority of Americans. You have chosen to change your life, and have taken action to do it. You have learned that life rewards action. Your reward is the new way you feel physically and mentally. Be excited, be happy – you deserve it today.

Be sure to write down how you feel about your weight loss and your accomplishment. Also, put in writing your goal for the next month. A good goal for next month is to increase your physical activity and to lose more weight while making your muscles more efficient. Over the next month, you will physically and mentally continue to lose additional fat tissue. Stay in touch as always, and if you have questions or need any advice, we're always here.

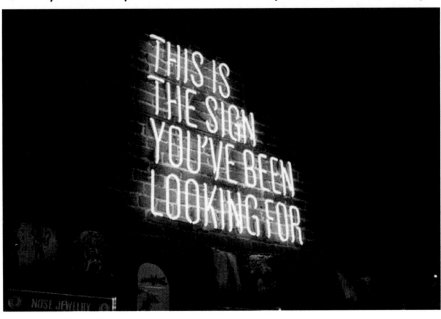

LEAN 51   DAILY TRACKER

Check off each item throughout the day to keep track of food, vitamins, water, and exercise.

Day # _____   Weight _____   Vitamin Pack _____

Your Daily Dietary Plan

Snack-Meal #1 _____   (Eat this first meal within 1 hour of arising)

Snack-Meal #2 _____

Snack-Meal #3 _____

Snack-Meal #4 _____

Snack-Meal #5 _____

Daily Fluid intake
each box equals 8oz.

Healthy Lean Meal   Protein   _____

2 Vegetables _____   Step Reading:_____

"Journaling is like whispering to one's self and listening at the same time."

~ Mina Murray

THE GOAL AND THE SOUL

Daily Goals

Write your goals in the space provided. These are your weight loss goals, your change-in-eating goals, your fitness and exercise goals and any other goals you want to achieve over time. Writing and re-writing goals daily is very powerful.

_____

_____

_____

_____

_____

_____

_____

Daily Soul
(Your Journal)

Write your feelings, thoughts and ideas below. These should include things you learned today, things you are excited about today, and things that you are grateful for today. Include any other details of the day you believe are important. This is your private workbook. Be honest with yourself. How do you really feel? Get it out of your head and on paper!

_____

_____

_____

_____

_____

_____

_____

What's Your Story
(Tasks and Victories)

_____

_____

_____

_____

_____

_____

_____

_____

_____

_____

"They are able because they think they are able."

~ Virgil

DAY 31
Metabolism

Lesson:

Our metabolism is the rate of our bodies' energy expenditure. It varies from one person to the next and is controlled by many factors. These factors include our age, current weight, genetics, diet, exercise, medical condition, thyroid status, and our muscle mass. Adjusting any of these factors will adjust our metabolic rate up or down.

Increasing exercise and increasing muscle mass in our body will raise our metabolism. If you feel that you have a slow metabolism, as many overweight people do, it can be evaluated through testing. In our office we can determine a person's calorie expenditure by using a device that determines oxygen consumption. Since oxygen is a required fuel to burn calories in our body, by measuring the body's consumption of oxygen we can calculate how many calories a person uses daily at rest, during normal activity, and with exercise.

This helps many of our patients understand how much food they can eat and why they've become overweight or obese in the first place. I encourage you to find a doctor who can measure this for you. If you cannot, let us know and we'll see if we can assist you in finding someone to measure your metabolism. Knowing how your body works is important in knowing how to feed it and treat it.

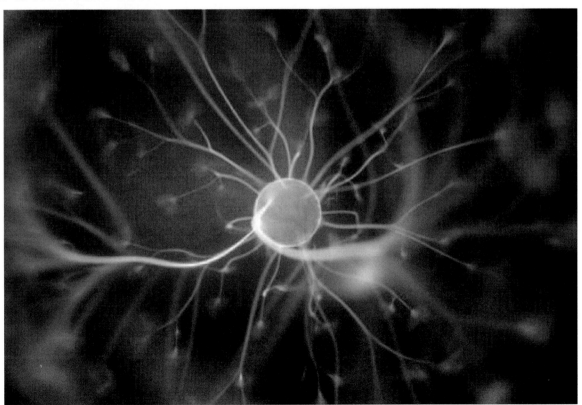

LEAN 51   DAILY TRACKER

Check off each item throughout the day to keep track of food, vitamins, water, and exercise.

Day # _____   Weight _____   Vitamin Pack _____

Your Daily Dietary Plan

Snack-Meal #1 _____   (Eat this first meal within 1 hour of arising)

Snack-Meal #2 _____

Snack-Meal #3 _____   ## Daily Fluid intake
                                  each box equals 8oz.

Snack-Meal #4 _____

Snack-Meal #5 _____

Healthy Lean Meal   Protein   _____

2 Vegetables _____   Step Reading:_____

"Journaling is like whispering to one's self and listening at the same time."

~ Mina Murray

THE GOAL AND THE SOUL

Daily Goals

Write your goals in the space provided. These are your weight loss goals, your change-in-eating goals, your fitness and exercise goals and any other goals you want to achieve over time. Writing and re-writing goals daily is very powerful.

_____

_____

_____

_____

_____

_____

_____

_____

Daily Soul
(Your Journal)

Write your feelings, thoughts and ideas below. These should include things you learned today, things you are excited about today, and things that you are grateful for today. Include any other details of the day you believe are important. This is your private workbook. Be honest with yourself. How do you really feel? Get it out of your head and on paper!

_____

_____

_____

_____

_____

_____

_____

What's Your Story
(Tasks and Victories)

_____

_____

_____

_____

_____

_____

_____

_____

_____

_____

"Walk boldly and wisely... There is a hand above that will help you on."

~ Phillip James Bailey

DAY 32
The Facts About Protein

Lesson:

Now that you're eating some protein 6 times a day, I thought a lesson on proteins would be helpful. Protein is one of the three essential elements known as macronutrients required for survival. The other two are fats and carbohydrates. The word "Protein" means "of prime importance." Each gram of protein gives your body four calories of energy potential.

Proteins are made up of chains of amino acids. Amino acids are the building blocks of our tissues. Proteins are important to build and maintain all of our muscles, our cells, our hormones, our antibodies for infection fighting and many transporters and communicator substances in our body.

Sources of dietary protein include animal and fish meats, plant products such as soybeans, legumes, nuts and seeds, as well as eggs and dairy products. If your diet is deficient in proteins, you will lose muscle mass, weaken your immunity and become unhealthy. If you eat too much protein, you will eventually convert the excess calories into fat tissue. On the LEAN 51 Program, you will get a healthy level of protein throughout the plan.

Proteins are digested and converted slowly to glucose, our major fuel source. A 4-6 ounce serving of protein takes about two hours for the body to fully process. The protein snack meals are strategically placed throughout the day to give you fuel and prevent cravings. Since you are "of prime importance" be sure to eat your proteins.

A dietary regimen, which leaves out a major nutrient group, cannot be healthful over a prolonged time period. You are learning how to use proteins, fats, and carbohydrates in a way that promotes life-long health. By eating proper quantities of each at the appropriate time, your body operates at peak performance. When your body is functioning at its peak level, you can perform at your peak level at home, at work, and at play.

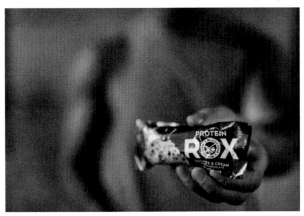

LEAN 51   DAILY TRACKER

Check off each item throughout the day to keep track of food, vitamins, water, and exercise.

Day # _____   Weight _____   Vitamin Pack _____

Your Daily Dietary Plan

Snack-Meal #1 _____   (Eat this first meal within 1 hour of arising)

Snack-Meal #2 _____

Snack-Meal #3 _____

Snack-Meal #4 _____

Snack-Meal #5 _____

Daily Fluid intake
each box equals 8oz.

Healthy Lean Meal   Protein   _____

2 Vegetables _____   Step Reading:_____

"Journaling is like whispering to one's self and listening at the same time."

~ Mina Murray

THE GOAL AND THE SOUL

Daily Goals

Write your goals in the space provided. These are your weight loss goals, your change-in-eating goals, your fitness and exercise goals and any other goals you want to achieve over time. Writing and re-writing goals daily is very powerful.

_____

_____

_____

_____

_____

_____

_____

Daily Soul
(Your Journal)

Write your feelings, thoughts and ideas below. These should include things you learned today, things you are excited about today, and things that you are grateful for today. Include any other details of the day you believe are important. This is your private workbook. Be honest with yourself. How do you really feel? Get it out of your head and on paper!

_____

_____

_____

_____

_____

_____

_____

<u>What's Your Story</u>
(Tasks and Victories)

_____

_____

_____

_____

_____

_____

_____

_____

_____

"Choosing a goal and sticking to it changes everything."

~ Scott Reed

DAY 33
Can Fat Be Important?

Lesson:

Though we are attempting to lose excess fat in our body, the groups of fats known as lipids do have importance to us. If you consume too much fat on a regular basis, your body will become too large and your health will deteriorate. Excess fat is associated with diabetes, heart and blood vessel disease, some cancers and a host of problems directly caused by obesity and the resultant increased body mass. The proper amount of fat and right kinds of fats are important to our normal body functions.

Fats are a source of stored energy. They keep us warm and serve as padding for protection. They help move some vitamins and medicines through our body and are necessary for certain hormone production such as estrogen and testosterone.

We now know that some fats, such as Omega-3 fatty acids are extremely beneficial, but usually deficient in the average American's diet. The Physicians Health Study revealed that men with the highest levels of Omega-3 fatty acids had an 80% lower chance of dying suddenly from cardiovascular events than men with the lowest levels!

On the LEAN 51 Program, you take 2 doses a day of high quality Omega 3 fatty acids derived from cold water fish. Incidentally, the most commonly consumed fish in the U.S. is catfish, which has no significant Omega-3 fatty acids. The good news is you are losing excess stored fat and eating healthier levels and types of fat on the LEAN 51 Program.

Once again, eating a proper balance of nutrients each day is the goal. Find a cold water fish that you enjoy eating and have it at least once a week. If you already eat fish 2-3 times weekly, you are ahead of the game. Do not skip your Omega-3 fatty acid supplements. When you run out, be sure to get more.

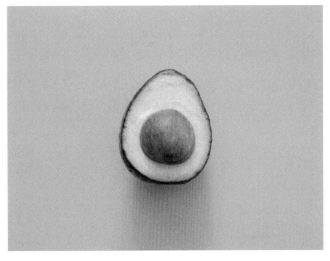

LEAN 51   DAILY TRACKER

Check off each item throughout the day to keep track of food, vitamins, water, and exercise.

Day # _____   Weight _____   Vitamin Pack _____

Your Daily Dietary Plan

Snack-Meal #1 _____   (Eat this first meal within 1 hour of arising)

Snack-Meal #2 _____

Snack-Meal #3 _____

Snack-Meal #4 _____

Snack-Meal #5 _____

Daily Fluid intake
each box equals 8oz.

Healthy Lean Meal   Protein   _____

2 Vegetables _____   Step Reading:_____

"Journaling is like whispering to one's self and listening at the same time."

~ Mina Murray

THE GOAL AND THE SOUL

Daily Goals

Write your goals in the space provided. These are your weight loss goals, your change-in-eating goals, your fitness and exercise goals and any other goals you want to achieve over time. Writing and re-writing goals daily is very powerful.

_____

_____

_____

_____

_____

_____

_____

Daily Soul
(Your Journal)

Write your feelings, thoughts and ideas below. These should include things you learned today, things you are excited about today, and things that you are grateful for today. Include any other details of the day you believe are important. This is your private workbook. Be honest with yourself. How do you really feel? Get it out of your head and on paper!

_____

_____

_____

_____

_____

_____

_____

What's Your Story
(Tasks and Victories)

_____

_____

_____

_____

_____

_____

_____

_____

_____

_____

_____

"Strong lives are motivated by dynamic purposes."

~ Kenneth Hildebrand

DAY 34
Picking Proteins

Lesson:

Since you need to eat a protein at each healthy meal, you need some variety to help from getting into the boredom rut. High quality proteins at a reasonable cost can be found on the following list.

- Ground beef, 85% lean or better
- Beef, top round
- Cheese, cheddar, low-fat if possible
- Cottage cheese, fat free
- Chicken breast, skinless
- Egg substitute
- Sliced lean ham
- Canadian bacon
- Low-fat cold cuts (98% fat free)
- Milk, skim or <1%
- Protein powders for shakes
- Protein cereals
- Whitish fish, i.e. cod, tilapia, scrod, lake, or ocean perch

- Salmon
- Tuna, white in water
- Turkey white
- Ground turkey
- Turkey, breast or tenderloins
- Lean pork, trim all fat
- Tofu, low fat
- String cheese, mozzarella
- Soybeans
- Soy Milk
- Non-fat yogurt
- Greek yogurt
- Whole egg

Now, don't you feel better about the variety of high quality proteins available as you continue to lose weight? Don't forget the protein snack meals either.

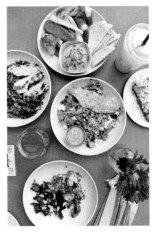

LEAN 51   DAILY TRACKER

Check off each item throughout the day to keep track of food, vitamins, water, and exercise.

Day # _____   Weight _____   Vitamin Pack _____

Your Daily Dietary Plan

Snack-Meal #1 _____   (Eat this first meal within 1 hour of arising)

Snack-Meal #2 _____

Snack-Meal #3 _____   **Daily Fluid intake**

Snack-Meal #4 _____   each box equals 8oz.

Snack-Meal #5 _____

Healthy Lean Meal   Protein   _____

              2 Vegetables _____   Step Reading:_____

"Journaling is like whispering to one's self and listening at the same time."

~ Mina Murray

THE GOAL AND THE SOUL

Daily Goals

Write your goals in the space provided. These are your weight loss goals, your change-in-eating goals, your fitness and exercise goals and any other goals you want to achieve over time. Writing and re-writing goals daily is very powerful.

_____

_____

_____

_____

_____

_____

_____

Daily Soul
(Your Journal)

Write your feelings, thoughts and ideas below. These should include things you learned today, things you are excited about today, and things that you are grateful for today. Include any other details of the day you believe are important. This is your private workbook. Be honest with yourself. How do you really feel? Get it out of your head and on paper!

_____

_____

_____

_____

_____

_____

_____

<u>What's Your Story</u>
(Tasks and Victories)

_____

_____

_____

_____

_____

_____

_____

_____

_____

_____

"Never bend your head. Hold it high. Look the world straight in the eye."

~ Helen Keller

DAY 35
Resistance Training

Lesson:

I know that the above title conjures up the thoughts of painful muscles, sprains, and the drudgery of pumping iron. Not on this program. If you dream is to look like Sylvester Stallone in Rambo or Jennifer Lopez in Enough, then go for it. Most of us just want to live leaner, longer, and healthier lives.

Toning your muscles is a great way to raise your fat burning capacity. You must start slow, be patient, and get some good advice. Resistance exercises are weight bearing exercises. Lifting a weight, pushing or pulling an object, or pressing against an opposing force constitutes resistance exercise. Recommendations from leading fitness trainers are to perform these exercises 2-3 days a week for 20-30 minutes each session.

Toning and increasing muscle mass, even slightly, will raise your metabolism, enhance your body's sensitivity to its own insulin and strengthen bones. One reason men typically lose weight faster than women, is due to their greater muscle mass. Most women aren't interested in building significant muscles since muscle does weigh more than fat, however, most women would like to have a tighter, leaner, fitter looking body. Check with your local gym, YMCA, YWCA or university for inexpensive instruction on resistance training. You'll be stronger for it.

A great rule to use when starting resistance training is the 10% rule. Start with a low amount of weight. This is weight you can lift or move easily. Perform approximately 10 repetitions of the exercise. After one week of using this weight and this number of repetitions, only increase either the weight or the repetitions in the second week by 10%. Continue to increase either weight or the repetitions in the second week by 10%. Alternate this process. It will seem slow at first, but will protect you from injury and muscle pain. Give it a try. You might find you like it.

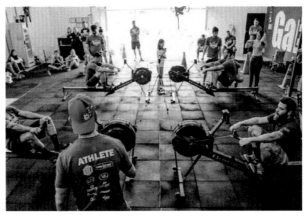

LEAN 51   DAILY TRACKER

Check off each item throughout the day to keep track of food, vitamins, water, and exercise.

Day # _____   Weight _____   Vitamin Pack _____

Your Daily Dietary Plan

Snack-Meal #1 _____   (Eat this first meal within 1 hour of arising)

Snack-Meal #2 _____

Snack-Meal #3 _____   **Daily Fluid intake**

each box equals 8oz.

Snack-Meal #4 _____

Snack-Meal #5 _____

Healthy Lean Meal   Protein   _____

2 Vegetables _____   Step Reading:_____

"Journaling is like whispering to one's self and listening at the same time."

~ Mina Murray

THE GOAL AND THE SOUL

Daily Goals

Write your goals in the space provided. These are your weight loss goals, your change-in-eating goals, your fitness and exercise goals and any other goals you want to achieve over time. Writing and re-writing goals daily is very powerful.

_____

_____

_____

_____

_____

_____

_____

Daily Soul
(Your Journal)

Write your feelings, thoughts and ideas below. These should include things you learned today, things you are excited about today, and things that you are grateful for today. Include any other details of the day you believe are important. This is your private workbook. Be honest with yourself. How do you really feel? Get it out of your head and on paper!

_____

_____

_____

_____

_____

_____

_____

What's Your Story
(Tasks and Victories)

_____

_____

_____

_____

_____

_____

_____

_____

_____

_____

"You don't live in a world all your own. Your brothers are here, too."

~ Albert Schweitzer

DAY 36
Setting the Example

Lesson:

This morning on CNN, I heard a specialist in Pediatric Endocrinology discussing the epidemic of childhood obesity and childhood diabetes. This professor from SUNY Medical College in Buffalo, NY stated that 42% of obese children have at least one obese parent. Obesity is now being diagnosed in children as young as 6 months of age with diabetes developing from obesity at age 2-1/2 years. We have an obligation to the future of this country to set an example for the children.

It doesn't matter whether you have children or not. Any one of us is a poor example if we ourselves are overweight. By the same token, any one of us is an example of health and vitality when we achieve our leaner, fitter body size. Sure, each of us started the LEAN 51 Program for our own health and well-being, but the power you will have to influence others is tremendous. You are part of a team of people that can change the health of a nation. I envision hundreds and then thousands of people with stories to tell about how they decid

ed to get healthy. We will walk together in local charity events. We will promote health as we touch lives day-to-day in our home, our work, our churches and our neighborhoods. You are a part of something big. You are part of something good. It may not feel like it, but you are a part of saving our nation's children.

Live Lean! Be the example!

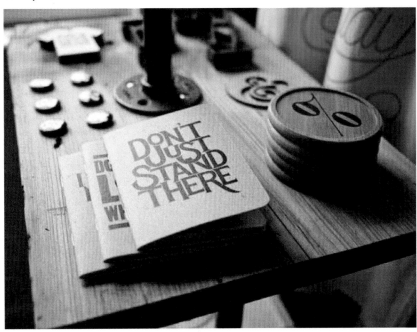

LEAN 51   DAILY TRACKER

Check off each item throughout the day to keep track of food, vitamins, water, and exercise.

Day # _____ Weight _____ Vitamin Pack _____

Your Daily Dietary Plan

Snack-Meal #1 _____ (Eat this first meal within 1 hour of arising)

Snack-Meal #2 _____

Snack-Meal #3 _____ **Daily Fluid intake**
each box equals 8oz.

Snack-Meal #4 _____

Snack-Meal #5 _____

Healthy Lean Meal   Protein   _____

2 Vegetables _____   Step Reading:_____

"Journaling is like whispering to one's self and listening at the same time."

~ Mina Murray

THE GOAL AND THE SOUL

Daily Goals

Write your goals in the space provided. These are your weight loss goals, your change-in-eating goals, your fitness and exercise goals and any other goals you want to achieve over time. Writing and re-writing goals daily is very powerful.

_____

_____

_____

_____

_____

_____

_____

Daily Soul
(Your Journal)

Write your feelings, thoughts and ideas below. These should include things you learned today, things you are excited about today, and things that you are grateful for today. Include any other details of the day you believe are important. This is your private workbook. Be honest with yourself. How do you really feel? Get it out of your head and on paper!

_____

_____

_____

_____

_____

_____

_____

What's Your Story
(Tasks and Victories)

_____

_____

_____

_____

_____

_____

_____

_____

_____

_____

"The only normal people are the ones you don't know very well."

~ Foe Ancis

DAY 37
Can You See Yourself?

Lesson:

No matter what your weight was when you started, you are now much closer to your ultimate goal. The question is "What is your ultimate goal?" Look at the goals you wrote when you painted a portrait of your future life. Are there any changes you want to make? How would you like to expand your vision?

Let me give you an example. I played athletics in school and stayed in great shape as long as I participated in sports. When this came to a halt, the weight started to pile on. I set a goal to walk my 10,000 steps a day and eventually I achieved that goal. I then reset a goal to go to the gym 6 days a week and attempt to jog a little. Later, I set an outrageous goal to jog for one hour without stopping. Ten months after I began my weight-loss program on Thanksgiving morning before the feast, I jogged 6-1/2 miles in one hour and felt great.

Don't be scared. You may never want to do something like that. The point is that you have accomplished great things in the past six weeks and you can accomplish anything you set your mind to. Visualize your future now and update your goals. Repaint your portrait of how you want to feel; what you want to look like; what your fitness level is; and how you want to live your life as a lean person. Set your goals, and visualize your future more confidently. Look ahead toward the direction of your dreams.

This is not a dress rehearsal. We don't get another chance to live life to the fullest. Continue to take personal responsibility for your health and your life. Don't become one of the heart disease and diabetes statistics. Never become too satisfied with how you are today. Life is ever changing and we cannot stand still. We are either getting better or losing ground.

I challenge you today to take what you have learned in the past six weeks on LEAN 51 and create a life that is truly inspiring to others. Inspire them with your commitment. Inspire them with your discipline. Inspire them with your vitality and your love of life. By reaching this part of the program, you have certainly inspired me. Set new goals and prepare to be an inspiration.

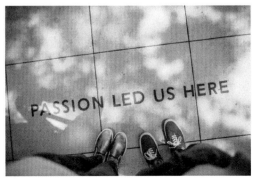

LEAN 51   DAILY TRACKER

Check off each item throughout the day to keep track of food, vitamins, water, and exercise.

Day # _____   Weight _____   Vitamin Pack _____

Your Daily Dietary Plan

Snack-Meal #1 _____   (Eat this first meal within 1 hour of arising)

Snack-Meal #2 _____

Snack-Meal #3 _____   **Daily Fluid intake**
each box equals 8oz.

Snack-Meal #4 _____

Snack-Meal #5 _____

Healthy Lean Meal   Protein   _____

2 Vegetables _____   Step Reading:_____

"Journaling is like whispering to one's self and listening at the same time."

~ Mina Murray

THE GOAL AND THE SOUL

Daily Goals

Write your goals in the space provided. These are your weight loss goals, your change-in-eating goals, your fitness and exercise goals and any other goals you want to achieve over time. Writing and re-writing goals daily is very powerful.

_____

_____

_____

_____

_____

_____

_____

Daily Soul
(Your Journal)

Write your feelings, thoughts and ideas below. These should include things you learned today, things you are excited about today, and things that you are grateful for today. Include any other details of the day you believe are important. This is your private workbook. Be honest with yourself. How do you really feel? Get it out of your head and on paper!

_____

_____

_____

_____

_____

_____

_____

What's Your Story
(Tasks and Victories)

_____

_____

_____

_____

_____

_____

_____

_____

_____

_____

"Friends are the sunshine of life."

~ John Hay

DAY 38
Heart Hospitals Everywhere

Lesson:

As a family physician in Indianapolis, IN, I often refer patients to heart specialists for specialized care. In the past few years, this city of approximately 1 ½-2 million people has opened several state of the art Heart Hospitals. There are five heart hospitals or cardiovascular centers in this one city. Why would this happen? From a doctor's view of the future, I know that diabetes is an epidemic, obesity is universal, and high blood pressure and elevated cholesterol are prevalent.

These cardiologists see the future and though they are intent on saving lives and helping people live healthier, they also know that billions of dollars will be spent correcting the heart damage and blood vessel damage associated with American's eating habits and sedentary behavior. Medicine's primary task is to serve, but it is also a business. Those doctors and hospitals with forward thinking are preparing to capitalize on the upcoming epidemic of heart disease, stroke, diabetes, and vascular disease. Don't you be a part of it. Keep doing what you're doing. Our goal on LEAN 51 is to help you stay out of these Heart Hospitals. Unfortunately, they will still do well without you. Tell a friend or loved one about your program. Maybe it will keep them out of these hospitals also.

Recently I attended a review of medicine conference given by the Harvard University Medical Center. A renowned Cardiologist at this prestigious center spoke to the large group of physicians. He spoke about cardiovascular health. He talked about the incredible medications and procedures currently being used to save lives.

The most profound statement he made, however, was that if individuals ate balanced diets, exercised regularly, and avoided smoking and excess alcohol, the need for these interventions could be reduced over 70%. These recommendations, if followed, would have more dramatic improvement in one's health than any of the currently available drugs or therapies on the market. Let LEAN 51 be the best insurance in your fight for heart and blood vessel health.

LEAN 51   DAILY TRACKER

Check off each item throughout the day to keep track of food, vitamins, water, and exercise.

Day # _____   Weight _____   Vitamin Pack _____

Your Daily Dietary Plan

Snack-Meal #1 _____   (Eat this first meal within 1 hour of arising)

Snack-Meal #2 _____

Snack-Meal #3 _____

Daily Fluid intake
each box equals 8oz.

Snack-Meal #4 _____

Snack-Meal #5 _____

Healthy Lean Meal   Protein   _____

2 Vegetables _____   Step Reading:_____

"Journaling is like whispering to one's self and listening at the same time."

~ Mina Murray

THE GOAL AND THE SOUL

Daily Goals

Write your goals in the space provided. These are your weight loss goals, your change-in-eating goals, your fitness and exercise goals and any other goals you want to achieve over time. Writing and re-writing goals daily is very powerful.

_____

_____

_____

_____

_____

_____

_____

Daily Soul
(Your Journal)

Write your feelings, thoughts and ideas below. These should include things you learned today, things you are excited about today, and things that you are grateful for today. Include any other details of the day you believe are important. This is your private workbook. Be honest with yourself. How do you really feel? Get it out of your head and on paper!

_____

_____

_____

_____

_____

_____

_____

<u>What's Your Story</u>
(Tasks and Victories)

_____

_____

_____

_____

_____

_____

_____

_____

_____

_____

"Having a goal is a state of happiness."

~ E. J. Bartek

DAY 39
Expand Your Success

Lesson:

You've proven that you can stick to a commitment. You've achieved success each and every day over the past 6-1/2 weeks. By following through on the LEAN 51 Program, and by losing weight, you have benefitted yourself in more ways than health improvement. You have enhanced your perception of yourself. You are stronger mentally and emotionally. Think of improving the other areas of your life the way you have your health.

Our lives can be segmented in what I call the 4 "F's" – Our faith, our family, our fitness, and our finances. You've done wonders toward improving your fitness. Keep at it for a lifetime. If you're like me and most other people, you probably would like to enhance your spiritual life or faith, whatever that may be. You most assuredly want the best family life and relationships you can have. I also bet you would enjoy greater financial fitness.

There is no secret to growing in the other areas of your life. Apply the same principles. Visualize what you want and paint a mental portrait of your future in each area. Write down your goals. Set a daily check off and task sheet to move closer each day to your goal. Track your progress by writing down measurable achievements.

Reward yourself for your accomplishments and encourage yourself when you slip. If you'd like to discuss these issues further, please feel free to e-mail. Several of us who want to enhance every part of our life work together and we help each other and hold each other accountable in the achievement of our goals in all four areas of our lives.

Just a thought for today!

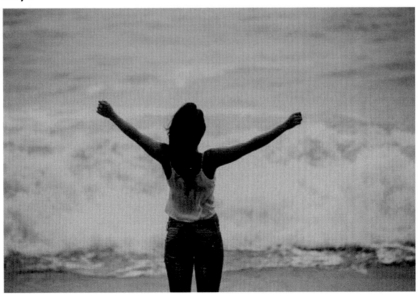

LEAN 51   DAILY TRACKER

Check off each item throughout the day to keep track of food, vitamins, water, and exercise.

Day # _____   Weight _____   Vitamin Pack _____

Your Daily Dietary Plan

Snack-Meal #1 _____   (Eat this first meal within 1 hour of arising)

Snack-Meal #2 _____

Snack-Meal #3 _____

Daily Fluid intake

each box equals 8oz.

Snack-Meal #4 _____

Snack-Meal #5 _____

Healthy Lean Meal   Protein   _____

2 Vegetables _____   Step Reading:_____

"Journaling is like whispering to one's self and listening at the same time."

~ Mina Murray

THE GOAL AND THE SOUL

Daily Goals

Write your goals in the space provided. These are your weight loss goals, your change-in-eating goals, your fitness and exercise goals and any other goals you want to achieve over time. Writing and re-writing goals daily is very powerful.

_____

_____

_____

_____

_____

_____

_____

Daily Soul
(Your Journal)

Write your feelings, thoughts and ideas below. These should include things you learned today, things you are excited about today, and things that you are grateful for today. Include any other details of the day you believe are important. This is your private workbook. Be honest with yourself. How do you really feel? Get it out of your head and on paper!

_____

_____

_____

_____

_____

<u>What's Your Story</u>
(Tasks and Victories)

"Doubt whom you will, but never yourself."

~ Christian Bovee

DAY 40
Body Reshape

Lesson:

Fat cells in our body can fill to a nice plump size. When they are getting larger, they stretch on surrounding tissues. Evaluation of our fat cells reveal that they are 90% filled with fat and 10% filled with water. As you lose fat, the cell will begin to temporarily change the ratio of fat and water. Initially, the cell keeps its large size and replaces lost fat with water. Hence, the additional water weight that is sometimes frustrating to the dieter. Over a few days, however, the water is reabsorbed and the cell shrinks, returning back to its 90% fat: 10% water ratio, this time at a smaller size.

LEAN 51 team members often notice a change in the way their body feels much sooner than people on other dietary programs. We believe that this rapid reduction in fat and preservation of muscle is the reason. On deprivation type diets, a person loses approximately 6.5 pounds of muscle tissue and 3.5 pounds of fat for every 10 pounds lost. Since this causes fatigue and weakness, it cannot be sustained.

With LEAN 51 you lose 9.5 pounds of fat and 0.5 pounds of muscle for every 10 pounds lost. These mechanisms promote continued energy and strength and gradually reshape your body to look leaner and become smaller in overall size. So, shape up!

In the United States, hundreds of billions of dollars are spent every year trying to improve the way we look. People undergo makeovers, style changes, take pills and so-called "fat burners" to attempt to look better and feel better about themselves. Many people resort to reconstructive or plastic surgery to change the way they look.

My recommendation is that before you subject yourself to painful permanent procedures, try LEAN 51 first. Reducing the fat and toning the muscle will not only make you feel great, but I know you'll feel better about yourself and your body. Each person is unique and special. Becoming all that we were meant to be is the greatest gift we can give to others.

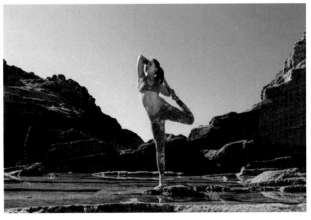

LEAN 51   DAILY TRACKER

Check off each item throughout the day to keep track of food, vitamins, water, and exercise.

Day # _____   Weight _____   Vitamin Pack _____

Your Daily Dietary Plan

Snack-Meal #1 _____   (Eat this first meal within 1 hour of arising)

Snack-Meal #2 _____

Snack-Meal #3 _____

Snack-Meal #4 _____

Snack-Meal #5 _____

Daily Fluid intake
each box equals 8oz.

Healthy Lean Meal   Protein   _____

2 Vegetables _____   Step Reading:_____

"Journaling is like whispering to one's self and listening at the same time."

~ Mina Murray

THE GOAL AND THE SOUL

Daily Goals

Write your goals in the space provided. These are your weight loss goals, your change-in-eating goals, your fitness and exercise goals and any other goals you want to achieve over time. Writing and re-writing goals daily is very powerful.

_____

_____

_____

_____

_____

_____

_____

Daily Soul
(Your Journal)

Write your feelings, thoughts and ideas below. These should include things you learned today, things you are excited about today, and things that you are grateful for today. Include any other details of the day you believe are important. This is your private workbook. Be honest with yourself. How do you really feel? Get it out of your head and on paper!

_____

_____

_____

_____

_____

_____

_____

<u>What's Your Story</u>
(Tasks and Victories)

_____

_____

_____

_____

_____

_____

_____

_____

_____

_____

"What isn't tried won't work."

~ Claude McDonald

DAY 41
Holidays and Special Events

Lesson:

Team members can become concerned when holidays and special events such as birthdays and weddings approach. We have always associated eating more with these special days. On LEAN 51 you don't have to worry. Take Thanksgiving as an example. The typical Thanksgiving Day meal includes a lean protein – white turkey.

A salad and a vegetable are always on the table that day. Fresh fruit or berries come in every cornucopia. On this day, you still get 100-150 grams of carbohydrates. Think it over in advance and decide which carbohydrates to choose from. If you must, select a small dish of mashed potatoes or a small dish of noodles. A dinner roll has 22 carbohydrate grams in it. Be selective.

Enjoy the feast by eating slowly. Close your eyes during the first few chews of each bite and savor the flavors. Enjoy the family and the conversation. Be grateful and thankful for the new healthier you. Get caught up in the spirit of the event and not the eating. Go for a walk before the meal and after the meal.

You may have eaten more on the holiday than your program days, but you did well and didn't gain any weight. Treat each holiday and special event the same way. Not only will they seem more special, but you will live to see so many more of them.

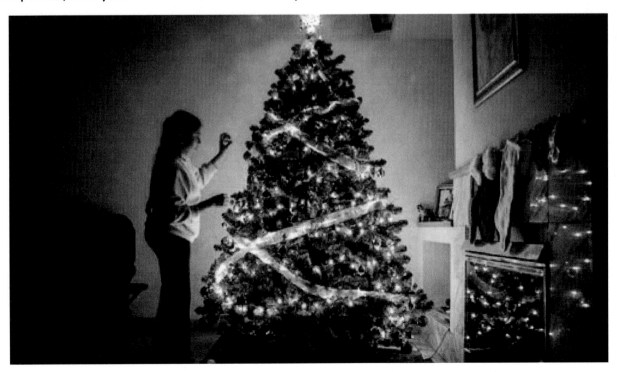

LEAN 51   DAILY TRACKER

Check off each item throughout the day to keep track of food, vitamins, water, and exercise.

Day # _____   Weight _____   Vitamin Pack _____

Your Daily Dietary Plan

Snack-Meal #1 _____   (Eat this first meal within 1 hour of arising)

Snack-Meal #2 _____

Snack-Meal #3 _____   **Daily Fluid intake**

Snack-Meal #4 _____   each box equals 8oz.

Snack-Meal #5 _____

Healthy Lean Meal   Protein   _____

2 Vegetables _____   Step Reading:_____

"Journaling is like whispering to one's self and listening at the same time."

~ Mina Murray

THE GOAL AND THE SOUL

Daily Goals

Write your goals in the space provided. These are your weight loss goals, your change-in-eating goals, your fitness and exercise goals and any other goals you want to achieve over time. Writing and re-writing goals daily is very powerful.

_____

_____

_____

_____

_____

_____

_____

Daily Soul
(Your Journal)

Write your feelings, thoughts and ideas below. These should include things you learned today, things you are excited about today, and things that you are grateful for today. Include any other details of the day you believe are important. This is your private workbook. Be honest with yourself. How do you really feel? Get it out of your head and on paper!

_____

_____

_____

_____

_____

_____

_____

What's Your Story
(Tasks and Victories)

_____

_____

_____

_____

_____

_____

_____

_____

_____

_____

"Courage to start and willingness to keep everlastingly at it are the requisites for success."

~ Alonzo Newton Benn

DAY 42
Not a Diet – A Lifelong Journey

Lesson:

When you began the LEAN 51 Program, you looked at it as another diet. By staying with the program through Day 42, you've realized it is more than a menu. You've figured out that a harsh diet, pills and muscle-fatiguing exercise is not needed to lose excess body fat and to feel better. You learned that the power to become healthy is within you. Though your family, friends, and doctor care about you, only you could make the decision to change your life. You have changed your life.

I know of no one who has spent six weeks on the program that doesn't feel stronger, more fit, and hasn't lost significant weight. For many, you will continue on the LEAN 51 Program for a month or two more. For a few, you will remain on the LEAN 51 Plan for many months until you reach your goal weight. The great news is that by completing 6 weeks, you know it can be done and that you have done it well to this point.

I know that you are aware of labels on foods. I know you understand the reasons for carbo-hydrate control and fat reduction. I know that you are more physically active and are doing things you couldn't have done only six weeks ago. I know your blood pressure is down and your cholesterol and lipids have improved. For those with medical problems, this may be a good time for a follow-up to let your physician know how well you are doing. You and your doctor can adjust therapies and treatments to fit your healthier body.

I encourage you to continue your progress toward complete health. Move toward your lean weight. Continue to have a life of abundance, energy, and happiness. When I say Live Lean, Live Long, and Live Life, it is more than just a slogan. It truly is a lifestyle and you are living it. I am here for you as you progress toward total health.

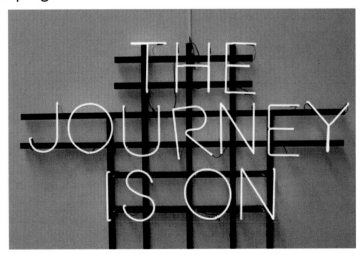

LEAN 51   DAILY TRACKER

Check off each item throughout the day to keep track of food, vitamins, water, and exercise.

Day # _____   Weight _____   Vitamin Pack _____

Your Daily Dietary Plan

Snack-Meal #1 _____   (Eat this first meal within 1 hour of arising)

Snack-Meal #2 _____

Snack-Meal #3 _____   **Daily Fluid intake**
                                  each box equals 8oz.

Snack-Meal #4 _____

Snack-Meal #5 _____

Healthy Lean Meal   Protein   _____

                      2 Vegetables _____   Step Reading:_____

"Journaling is like whispering to one's self and listening at the same time."

~ Mina Murray

THE GOAL AND THE SOUL

Daily Goals

Write your goals in the space provided. These are your weight loss goals, your change-in-eating goals, your fitness and exercise goals and any other goals you want to achieve over time. Writing and re-writing goals daily is very powerful.

_____

_____

_____

_____

_____

_____

Daily Soul
(Your Journal)

Write your feelings, thoughts and ideas below. These should include things you learned today, things you are excited about today, and things that you are grateful for today. Include any other details of the day you believe are important. This is your private workbook. Be honest with yourself. How do you really feel? Get it out of your head and on paper!

_____

_____

_____

_____

_____

_____

_____

What's Your Story
(Tasks and Victories)

_____

_____

_____

_____

_____

_____

_____

_____

_____

_____

"If you wish success in life, make perseverance your bosom friend."

~ Joseph Addison

DAY 43
Personal Improvement

Lesson:

Though I have never met him, Brian Tracey is a mentor of mine. I have read all his books and studied all of his programs. He believes that any person can achieve anything they desire by following a pattern of daily self-improvement. By finding one small thing each day that can improve yourself and working on that, you can quickly become excellent at that thing.

Over the past 43 days, you have done this. You have recorded your goals and aspirations each day. You have found new ways to stay on the program. You have learned from others who have gone before you on the LEAN 51 Program. You increased your physical exercise day by day through the step program.

This daily self-improvement is the essence of success. Your success with weight loss has been because of your constant work to change the bad habits of your life and replace them with good healthful habits. Continue to write your goals daily. Continue to challenge yourself with new goals.

Never settle for feeling comfortable. Stretch yourself. Stretch your thinking. Stretch your body's capabilities. Continue to grow into your best self. As you continue living the LEAN life-style, work hard to make this your best year yet. Be sure to look back at your goals and reflect on your achievements. Then set new goals immediately. Strive for constant and never-ending improvement.

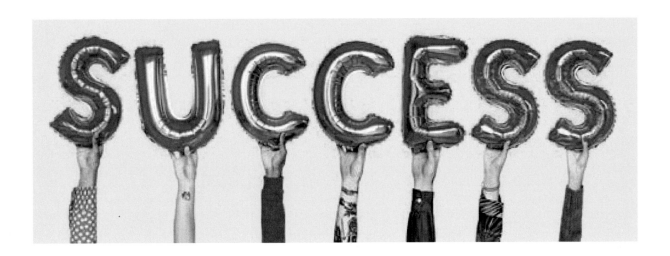

LEAN 51   DAILY TRACKER

Check off each item throughout the day to keep track of food, vitamins, water, and exercise.

Day # _____   Weight _____   Vitamin Pack _____

Your Daily Dietary Plan

Snack-Meal #1 _____   (Eat this first meal within 1 hour of arising)

Snack-Meal #2 _____

Snack-Meal #3 _____   **Daily Fluid intake**
each box equals 8oz.

Snack-Meal #4 _____

Snack-Meal #5 _____

Healthy Lean Meal   Protein   _____

2 Vegetables _____   Step Reading:_____

"Journaling is like whispering to one's self and listening at the same time."

~ Mina Murray

THE GOAL AND THE SOUL

Daily Goals

Write your goals in the space provided. These are your weight loss goals, your change-in-eating goals, your fitness and exercise goals and any other goals you want to achieve over time. Writing and re-writing goals daily is very powerful.

_____

_____

_____

_____

_____

_____

_____

Daily Soul
(Your Journal)

Write your feelings, thoughts and ideas below. These should include things you learned today, things you are excited about today, and things that you are grateful for today. Include any other details of the day you believe are important. This is your private workbook. Be honest with yourself. How do you really feel? Get it out of your head and on paper!

_____

_____

_____

_____

_____

What's Your Story
(Tasks and Victories)

"The reward of a thing well done is to have done it."

~ Ralph Waldo Emerson

DAY 44
Completion

Lesson:

Today is a milestone for you. You have completed 6 weeks of LEAN 51. Congratulations! If you are now at your lean weight, you are ready for the Maintenance Program. If you have additional fat to lose, continue to follow the program and work with your coach. Repeat your daily plan until you reach your goal weight. When you are at your goal weight, move to the Maintenance Plan, which your coach will work with you on.

You have learned to eat properly to reach your lean weight. You can return to the LEAN 51 weight loss plan anytime you experience a 5-pound weight gain. You have learned to increase your body movement and to raise your metabolism. You have learned to think more positively and visualize your future.

You have set an example for your loved ones, your neighbors, your friends, your co-workers and all that you come in contact with. You are painting a new portrait each day of how you want to live your life. You have helped us expand our vision and you are not just a client or a patient, you are a friend. You are now trained to Live Lean, Live Long, Live Life and Spread the Health!

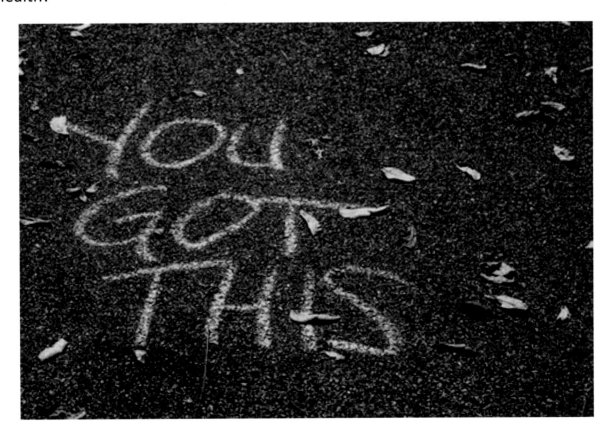

LEAN 51   DAILY TRACKER

Check off each item throughout the day to keep track of food, vitamins, water, and exercise.

Day # _____   Weight _____   Vitamin Pack _____

Your Daily Dietary Plan

Snack-Meal #1 _____   (Eat this first meal within 1 hour of arising)

Snack-Meal #2 _____

Snack-Meal #3 _____   **Daily Fluid intake**

each box equals 8oz.

Snack-Meal #4 _____

Snack-Meal #5 _____

Healthy Lean Meal   Protein   _____

2 Vegetables _____   Step Reading:_____

"Journaling is like whispering to one's self and listening at the same time."

~ Mina Murray

THE GOAL AND THE SOUL

Daily Goals

Write your goals in the space provided. These are your weight loss goals, your change-in-eating goals, your fitness and exercise goals and any other goals you want to achieve over time. Writing and re-writing goals daily is very powerful.

_____

_____

_____

_____

_____

_____

_____

Daily Soul
(Your Journal)

Write your feelings, thoughts and ideas below. These should include things you learned today, things you are excited about today, and things that you are grateful for today. Include any other details of the day you believe are important. This is your private workbook. Be honest with yourself. How do you really feel? Get it out of your head and on paper!

_____

_____

_____

_____

_____

What's Your Story
(Tasks and Victories)

Weight Maintenance

You have now reached a weight where you feel great, look great, and are healthy. Many of the present or potential medical issues due to excess body fat have been eliminated or the risk is much less due to your efforts. The key now is to continue to live a lean and healthy life for good.

If you have not reached your desired weight, just continue on the LEAN 51 plan as in the first 44 days. Feel free to copy any Tracker sheets and Journaling pages to assist in your ongoing plan.

If you are now at your goal weight, it is important to find out how many calories you can consume daily to maintain this new lean body. A good estimate to maintain a healthy weight is to eat about 2000 calories per day for women and about 2500 calories daily for men. Another more precise method is to calculate your current body weight in kilograms. (2.2 pounds/kilogram) Next, multiply the number of kilograms by 24. This will give you a close caloric daily intake for weight stability. Example: 170 pounds/2.2 = 72 kilograms. 72 X 24 = 1,728 calories per day.

Certainly there are varying circumstances for each person and if you find that your weight goes up on this number of calories a day, you must reduce that number until you reach a state of weight equilibrium. If your weight continues to fall, you must add some calories to each day until body weight stabilizes.

Anytime you regain more than 5% of your current healthy body weight return to the LEAN 51 plan until you have returned to your goal weight.

Feel free to contact Dr. Oliver or a coach with any questions through one of the following methods:

Facebook: fastclinicalweightloss   **Email: FatDocThinDoc@gmail.com**

LinkedIN: Greg Oliver

For additional info and tips, see our daily FB or LinkedIN posts

Podcast: The Skinny with Fat Doc and Malibu Macie

Website: FastClinicalWeightLoss.com

Maintenance

You've Reached Your Healthy Weight!
Follow The 8 Simple <u>Maintain</u> Steps Bellow to Be Healthy For Life!

M	**MENU** -- follow it daily
A	**ACTIVITY**-- daily intentional physical activity/exercise
I	**INITIAL MEAL OF THE DAY** -- consumed within 1 hour of waking
N	**NOTE WELL** - journal your goals & soul daily
T	**TEACH** others how to be healthy
A	**ACCOUNTABILITY** -- stay in touch with your Health Coach
I	**INTERVAL EATING** -- eat meals and snackmeals every 2 $\frac{1}{2}$ - 3 hours
N	**NEVER ALLOW A WEIGHT GAIN OVER 5%** of your body weight without contacting your Health Coach to restart your weight loss plan

MAINTENANCE MENU

Start eating within 1 hour of rising
space eating every 2 $\frac{1}{2}$ - 3 hours

Breakfast
1 protein serving (4-6 oz)
1 grain serving
1 fruit serving
1 zero calorie beverage

Morning Snackmeal

Lunch
1 protein serving
2 vegetable servings
1 zero calorie beverage

Afternoon Snackmeal

Dinner
1 protein serving (4-6 oz.)
2 vegetable servings
1 fruit or grain serving
1 zero calorie beverage

Evening Snackmeal

*If you gain weight or continue to lose weight on this menu plan,
contact your Health Coach for modification.

Healthy Food Options

Protein: 4-6 oz servings
Grilled, baked, broiled, or poached - not fried

Fish	Lean Pork	Egg Whites	98% Lean Cold Cuts
Shellfish	Lean Beef	Egg Beaters	Game Meats
Tuna	Veggie Burger	Turkey	Lamb
Tofu	Fat Free cheese	Chicken	Low Fat Cottage cheese

Vegetable: Serving = 1 Cup

Celery	Cabbage	Mixed Veggies	Broccoli	Kohlrabi	Squash
Okra	Sprouts	Asparagus	Onions	Lettuce	kale
Turnips	Tomatoes	Cauliflower	Peppers	Spinach	Greens
Radishes	Mushrooms	Green Beans	Cucumber	Salad	

Fruits: 1 serving = small piece of fruits or 1/2 cup

Apple	½ Banana	Nectarine	Cantaloupe	Tomato	Peach
Pear	Apricots	Tangerine	Dates	Grapes	Plums
Orange	Mango	Papaya	Kiwi	Berries	Melon

Grains

Whole Grain Bread: 1 Slice	1 Tortilla (low carb/whole grain): 1 tortilla
Cereal (no added sugar): 1/2 - 2/4 cup	English muffin: 1/2 English Muffin

Condiments
> 1 Tablespoon of mustard or ketchup
> Dill pickles
> Herbal and natural seasonings

Healthy Fats
> 2 Tablespoons of regular or low-carb dressing
> 1 teaspoon of margarine
> 1 teaspoon of Olive Oil

Beverage
> 64 oz. of water
> Any zero calorie liquids

Conclusion

Frequently Asked Questions

Q: Can anyone be on the LEAN 51 Program?

A: Almost everyone can utilize the LEAN 51 Program. As a physician I don't recommend this or any other weight loss program to A) Women who are pregnant or breast-feeding, B) Patients with any severe disease process or organ damage, C) Patients with Type I, insulin dependent (previously juvenile diabetes) diabetes. Adolescents can be on the program. We place them on a modified plan. This is not a medically prescribed program. It is a safe, healthy way to eat and achieve your lean body weight.

Q: Is this like the Atkins diet?

A: No. The Atkins diet is a high protein, high fat, very low or no carbohydrate program. LEAN 51 is a normal protein, reduced carbohydrate (approx. 100-150 grams/day) controlled fat program.

Q: Can I substitute items on the plan?

A: If you modify the plan, you may not lose the weight. The program is designed to give you the proper nutrients at the proper time and supplements to support that. Any changes may alter your progress. I have had several people change the snack-meals, the menus and the supplements only to come back frustrated. When they followed the plan closely, they were very pleased and reached their goal.

Q: What if I don't live near one of your weight loss clinics?

A: This program comes in a complete, self-explanatory kit. The kit and any materials can be shipped anywhere in the country or Canada. You can participate by e-mail or stay in touch through our websites.

Q: Do I have to do strenuous workouts?

A: No. This program is designed to increase your physical activity through step-tracked walking program. See the chapter on the walking plan.

Q: Can children be on the LEAN 51 Plan?

A: Children over 12 are put on a modified, higher calorie plan. They require more protein and more calories to give them the required nutrients for growth. Since this plan is very balanced and provides for all nutrients, it is safe for adolescents and teens. For children less than 12 years old, consult with their pediatrician or family doctor.

Q: Do I have to buy or eat packaged food?

A: No, you will be obtaining your food for your healthy meal or meals from your local grocer. The nutritional snack-meals and supplements are available through our clinics or at fastclinicalweightloss.com

Q: Can I drink alcoholic beverages on LEAN 51?

A: I always say, "Yes, but you won't lose any weight." During the LEAN 51 program, avoid alcoholic beverages. In the maintenance phase, limited amounts can be counted as carbohydrates. Some new beers are available with reduced carbohydrates. Remember, however, that alcoholic beverages are essentially excess calories.

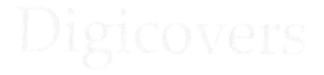

Real People – Real Results

David - David is the typical 18-year old student who spends a great deal of time doing homework, meeting with friends, and using the computer. Today's teens get much less physical activity unless they are participating in athletics. Over time, the reduced activity and the high carbohydrate, high fat diet of teenagers took its toll on David.

He gained a significant amount of weight. When he began the program, his goal was to be in better shape for spring break of his senior year in high school. He worked at the program and lost 30 pounds in three months. He told me that he liked the snack meals and felt he couldn't always eat the volume of food on the program. Today David has lost a total of 68 pounds and is approaching his ideal weight. He went from 271 pounds to 203 pounds. He is on maintenance and has developed much healthier eating habits.

Mark - Mark is who I call, the "Poster Child" for the LEAN 51 program. Mark began the program at 388 pounds. He has lost 160 pounds in 15 months and is now working to achieve his optimal weight of 198 pounds. Mark lives the program and has become a coach. He works with others to answer questions and give advice from his acquired wealth of personal experience. Mark has added years to his life and energy to his days. He continues to set goals and work toward improvement in all areas of his life.

Paula - Paula is a patient of mine who is a delight to work with. I wouldn't let Paula start the program until I worked through it myself. She asked me every month if she could start. I finally placed her on the plan and she has lost 90 pounds. She has reduced medication for her blood pressure and is becoming the picture of health. She recently set a goal to walk a 13.1-mile Mini-Marathon and she thrilled us by completing it in a very impressive time. Paula is an inspiration to many of us. She truly is a star.

Glenda - Glenda has lost 100 pounds on the program. She is always upbeat and excited about life. She knows her carbs and she understands the importance of snack meals. Glenda attributes her incredible achievement to eating every 3 hours. She follows a progressive walking program and counts her steps daily with her step tracker. I believe she has worn out a tracker or two. Having Glenda on the team adds to the fun as she is one of the most positive people I know.

Rebecca - Rebecca joined the plan and reached her optimal weight with a 50-pound weight loss. She worked until her goal was met. Her son came to our office with her and related that when he returned home from college for summer break, he hardly recognized his mom. Rebecca looks 10-15 years younger in her lean, fit body. She lives the program daily and has inspired many of her co-workers to begin the plan. I salute her for a job well done.

Live Lean, Live Long, Live Life

The above slogan was coined as several of us moved through the LEAN 51 Program. As time went on, the phrase took on greater meaning. When people dropped enough weight to see their cholesterol improve or their blood pressure drop, the slogan came alive. Our team members were truly improving their health, extending their lives, and enjoying themselves along the journey. Throughout history, many have repeated the saying "If you don't' have your health, you don't have anything." We all realize this is true, but, we tend to suppress it as we go through life eating, drinking, and gaining weight.

I challenge you as a team member to help someone else take the same journey you've been on. You don't even have to confront someone about their health or their weight issues. You only have to be a daily living example of what it means to Live Lean, Live Long, Live Life.

I wish you well, I wish you good health, and I wish you the life you painted in your mental portrait.

Our Mission

"Spread the Health"

1. Become Healthy on LEAN 51.
2. Encourage a friend or family member to join you.
3. Create a team of achievers.
4. Become the change you wish to see in our community, our country, and the world

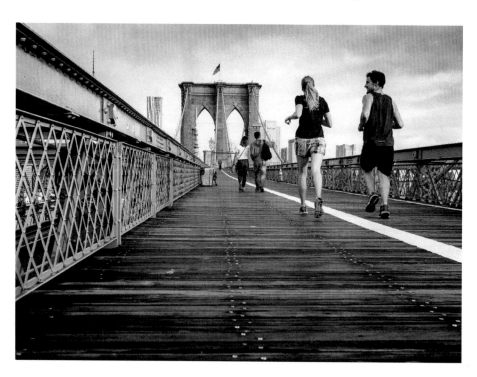

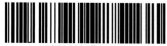

53653035R00117

Made in the USA
Columbia, SC
18 March 2019